HOME
*A*ROMATHERAPY

A step-by-step guide on using essential oils at home

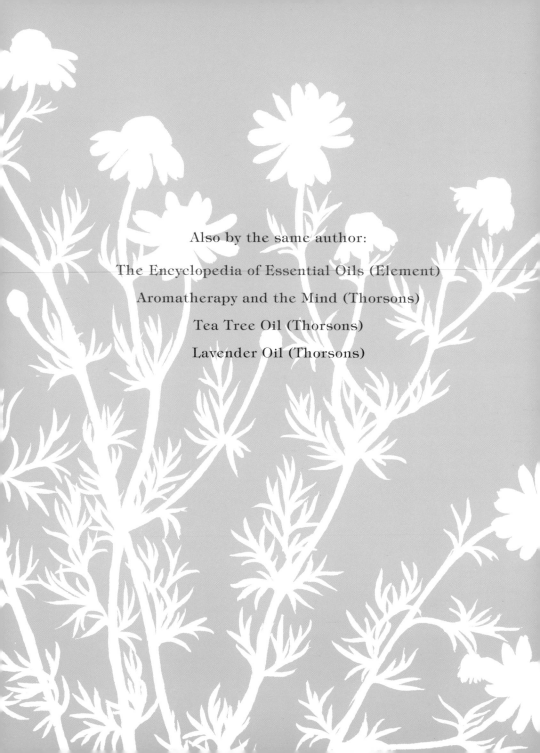

Also by the same author:

The Encyclopedia of Essential Oils (Element)

Aromatherapy and the Mind (Thorsons)

Tea Tree Oil (Thorsons)

Lavender Oil (Thorsons)

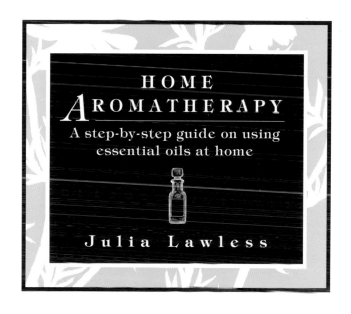

HOME
AROMATHERAPY

A step-by-step guide on using
essential oils at home

Julia Lawless

Illustrations by
Sally Maltby

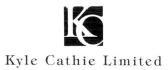

Kyle Cathie Limited

First published in Great Britain 1993 by
Kyle Cathie Limited
7/8 Hatherley Street
London SW1P 2QT

Reprinted 1994

This edition 1995

ISBN 1 85626 174 3

Julia Lawless is hereby identified as the author of this work in accordance
with Section 77 of the Copyright, Designs and Patents Act 1988

A Cataloguing in Publication record for this title is available from
the British Library

Designed by Lisa Steffens

Printed and bound in Hong Kong

Cover illustration of *German chamomile* (Matricaria recutica).

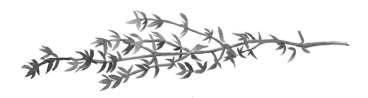

CONTENTS

To Len

ACKNOWLEDGEMENTS

I would first like to thank Chris and Sarah Moreland whose inspiration gave form to this book; Alex, Chiara and Anna for supporting my involvement with essential oils over the years; Ute and Myles for their help, especially over weekends; my mother Kerttu, whose lifelong fascination for herbs and aromatics inspired me, even as a child; Kyle and Beverley at Kyle Cathie Limited and Sally Maltby, the illustrator, for being such a pleasure to work with on this project; as well as my husband Alec and daughter Natasha for their assistance, in all sorts of ways, during the writing of this book.

I would also especially like to thank my father, to whom this book is dedicated, for encouraging me to write a 'lay person's' guide to the use of essential oils based on my own experience. This book, consequently, has a very personal flavour. For example, I tend to use *lavender* for virtually all first-aid requirements in the home, especially for my daughter – and this is reflected in the text. Together with *chamomile* and *tea tree*, these are the three essential oils I would never be without. When it comes to the more pleasurable side of aromatics, I find my preferences change according to mood, although *rose*, *jasmine* and *neroli* are always high on the list.

I have not set out to break new ground with this book, nor have I attempted to cover all the essential oils which are now available. I have simply tried to select those oils which I find to be the most useful – other less common oils such as *cinnamon leaf*, *camphor*, *hyssop* or *coriander* are not what I would consider *essential* for home use. What I do hope this book achieves is to provide a straightforward and inspiring guide for all who are interested in 'home aromatherapy', a guide which is both simple and pleasurable to use.

AN INTRODUCTION TO AROMATHERAPY

What is Aromatherapy?

Aromatherapy is a form of healing that utilizes the natural aromatic aspect of plants – the essential oils – both for their scent and for their inherent medicinal properties. These aromatic oils can be found in a wide range of species and are extracted (usually by steam distillation) from the seeds, bark, leaves, flowers, wood, roots or resin according to the type of plant. The bitter orange tree, for example, produces *orange* oil from the fruit, *petitgrain* oil from the leaves and *neroli* or *orange blossom* oil from the flowers – each one has a very distinct character.

The term 'aromathérapie' was first coined in the 1920s by the French perfumier René Gattefossé, who became involved in extensive research into the medicinal properties of aromatic oils after discovering, by accident, that *lavender* oil was able to speed up the healing process of a severe burn and prevent scarring. When in 1928 he published a book of that name describing his discoveries, he re-ignited interest in what is essentially a long-standing healing tradition.

For although the word 'aromatherapy' is new, the knowledge and use of aromatics and essential oils for healing purposes reaches back to the very heart of the earliest civilizations. Aromatic oils and unguents, for example, were employed by the ancient Egyptians some four thousand years ago. The Greek and Roman culture was renowned for its emphasis on the benefits of aromatic bathing and adornment, while the Chinese and Indian traditions still use aromatics extensively as part of their herbal medical system, as well as for ritual purposes. It was only during the last century in the West that the use of home remedies (including natural aromatics) underwent a decline as a result of the scientific revolution and the development of the modern drug industry.

The practice and art of aromatherapy has stood the test of time. Over the last decade it has enjoyed an ever increasing popularity, reflecting the general trend towards 'holistic' types of therapy (which aim to treat the 'whole' person) and a growing preference for natural products that are environmentally friendly.

How Does it Work?

The word 'aromatherapy' can be misleading, because it suggests a type of healing which operates simply through our sense of smell. This is not true. The fragrance of essential oils is an important part of their overall nature, but only one aspect of it.

In an aromatherapy treatment, essential oils interact with the body in a variety of ways. When a massage oil is prepared with essential oils and rubbed on to the skin, the essential oils are quickly absorbed through the cell tissue and into the bloodstream to be transported throughout the body. They can then interact with the organs and systems of the body directly – some, such as *chamomile* or *lavender*, may sedate the nervous system; some may stimulate the circulation, like *rosemary* or *black pepper*; while others, like *fennel* or *juniper*, have a detoxifying or purifying effect on the blood.

Massage is the main method used by professional aromatherapists because it ensures a good absorption of the essential oils and is a very relaxing and healing experience in itself. The oils are also absorbed into the body when they are mixed with creams or facial lotions. They are ideally suited to skin care, because they not only act 'on site' but also penetrate deep beneath the skin's surface, helping to eliminate the problem at its source. The application of *chamomile* oil to an infected sore, for example, can help prevent inflammation and pain and speed up the healing process by increasing cell regeneration.

Essential oils are not greasy like vegetable oils, they are volatile liquids that easily evaporate into the air without leaving a trace behind. When oils are used in the bath, a certain amount is absorbed through the

8

skin and the rest is diffused into the air. Hot water, or the presence of any type of heat, encourages them to evaporate more quickly than they do at room temperature. When essential oils are inhaled they are carried into the lungs and a proportion is absorbed via the alveoli into the blood. Vaporized essential oils are actually absorbed into the bloodstream faster than if they had been taken orally – a method which is best avoided! The practice of vaporizing oils using an oil burner or diffuser is particularly useful for respiratory infections or contagious diseases.

In addition, essential oils act on our emotional and mental states through their fragrances. Our sense of smell is closely linked to our feelings and memories – for example, a specific odour can instantly conjure up our associations with a particular place or experience. Two olfactory nerve tracts run straight into the limbic system of the brain, which is concerned with memory and emotion, bypassing the central nervous system. This means that a smell can have an immediate and powerful effect that defies rational analysis.

Our response to different scents is very individual, but there is no doubt that perfumes can help to evoke different moods and create a particular type of atmosphere. This is why incense is used in religious and ritual practices all over the world. *Frankincense*, for example, is employed by the Roman Catholic Church and could be said to create a meditative mood, whereas *patchouli* oil, which is extensively used to scent cloth in India, brings with it the sensual atmosphere of the East.

The emotive fragrances of aromatic oils are thus combined with their physiological effect as they interact with the systems of the body. In this way, an aromatherapy treatment could be seen to work on a variety of different levels, where the physical and the emotional, the body and the mind, are both brought into play. It is this combination of factors that accounts for the success aromatherapy enjoys in reducing stress (see page 31), which is at the root of so many of our modern complaints.

By employing different methods of application, aromatherapy can thus be used to deal effectively with a wide range of common conditions, including skin problems such as acne, eczema and fungal conditions;

respiratory disorders like coughs, bronchitis and sinusitis; rheumatism and arthritis; muscular aches and pains; as well as nervous and emotional difficulties. Some complaints, especially of a chronic or long-standing nature, are best dealt with in a professional context, but one of the greatest pleasures of essential oils is that they can also be used simply, safely and effectively in the home.

Essential Oils and their Properties

Each essential oil is made up of a unique and complex blend of chemical constituents that define its particular character. *Eucalyptus* oil, for example, contains a large proportion of a substance called 'cineol' or 'eucalyptol' which gives *eucalyptus* its familiar camphoraceous odour. Cineol is an excellent antiseptic and expectorant, it kills germs, and it loosens and expels mucus, which is why *eucalyptus* is such a useful oil for coughs, colds and general congestion. Other camphoraceous oils which are high in cineol, such as *tea tree*, *marjoram* and *rosemary*, consequently share similar properties and are also used for respiratory infection. Indeed, most essential oils stimulate the immune system, encourage the body's innate curative powers and have bactericidal properties.

Lavender, which is a particularly versatile oil, contains a large amount of a constituent called 'linalyl acetate' which has a sedative effect and which gives *lavender* its fruity, sweet quality. *Lavender* also contains some cineol, which accounts for its antiseptic and expectorant action. There are several major constituents in *lavender* which each have their own properties, as well as many minor constituents and trace elements that all contribute to its overall character. This is why it is very difficult to synthesize or imitate a natural essential oil in the laboratory – *rose* oil, for example, includes over three hundred different constituents.

German chamomile oil (and *roman chamomile* to a lesser degree) contains an important constituent called 'chamazulene' that accounts for its inky blue colour and its outstanding anti-inflammatory, wound-healing and soothing properties. *Roman chamomile* (and *german chamomile* to a lesser degree) contains a large proportion of 'esters', which in addition have a sedative or relaxing effect. In a condition such as eczema, where the manifestation of a skin rash is often connected with an underlying emotional upset, the multi-faceted properties of *chamomile* are able to address both problems simultaneously.

Many essential oils have a variety of properties. An oil such as *bergamot* is soothing to the nervous system, yet uplifting to the mind; a regulating oil such as *geranium* is either relaxing or reviving according to the individual's need. Other oils like *patchouli* can be stimulating in small amounts but sedating or even soporific in excess – much like wine!

The following list is by no means complete, but provides a good basis for understanding each oil's potential:

Stimulating Oils
(for low blood pressure and lack of energy):
Basil, black pepper, cardomon, ginger, peppermint, pine needle, rosemary, thyme.

Relaxing Oils
(for emotional or physical tension):
Atlas cedarwood, bergamot, chamomile, clary sage, cypress, frankincense, jasmine, lavender, marjoram, neroli, rose, sandalwood, vetiver, ylang ylang.

Expectorant Oils
(for colds, coughs and congestion):
Eucalyptus, myrtle, peppermint, pine needle, rosemary, spanish sage, thyme.

Antiseptic Oils
(for any kind or virus or infection):
Basil, bergamot, clary sage, clove, eucalyptus, fennel, lavender, lemon, pine needle, rosemary, spanish sage, tea tree, thyme.

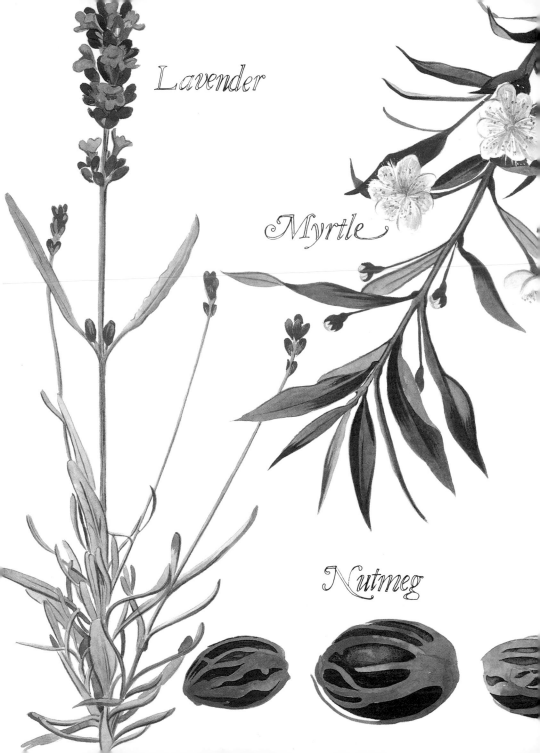

Lavender

Myrtle

Nutmeg

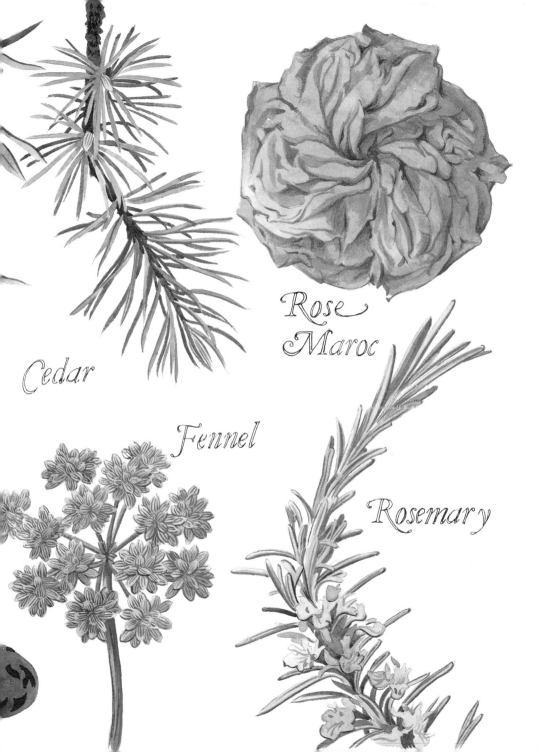

Cedar

Rose
Maroc

Fennel

Rosemary

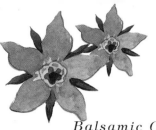

Balsamic Oils

(to soothe irritating coughs or bronchitis):
Atlas cedarwood, benzoin, cypress, frankincense, juniper, pine needle, sandalwood.

Detoxifying/Cleansing Oils

(for cellulitis, skin eruptions, arthritis, etc.):
Carrot seed, cypress, fennel, grapefruit, hyssop, juniper, lemon, mandarin, orange, thyme.

Anti-inflammatory/Healing Oils

(for infected cuts, sores, stings, etc.):
Benzoin, bergamot, chamomile, frankincense, geranium, lavender, myrrh, palmarosa, patchouli, rose.

Anti-spasmodic Oils

(for period pains, indigestion, muscular cramps, etc.):
Black pepper, cardomon, chamomile, clary sage, fennel, ginger, jasmine, lavender, marjoram, nutmeg, orange, pine needle, rosemary.

Anti-depressant Oils

(for post-natal depression, listlessness, etc.):
Basil, benzoin, bergamot, geranium, jasmine, lavender, neroli, petitgrain, rose, ylang ylang.

Aphrodisiac Oils

(to increase sexual desire):
Black pepper, cardomon, ginger, jasmine, myrtle, neroli, nutmeg, patchouli, rose, rosewood, sandalwood, ylang ylang.

Insect Repellents

Atlas cedarwood, basil, citronella, clove, eucalyptus, geranium, lavender, lemongrass, myrtle, patchouli, peppermint, thyme.

Methods of Use

BATH

This is the easiest and most popular way of using essential oils at home. Simply add 5–10 drops of a chosen oil to the bath water when the tub is full and relax in the aromatic vapours. Different essential oils can be selected for their specific effect – for example, *rosemary* is reviving and stimulating, *chamomile* is soothing and relaxing. The oils can be blended together for bathing, but take care not to exceed 10 drops in total.

Essential oils can also be mixed in a teaspoon of vegetable oil (such as sweet almond oil) before being added to the bath. This helps to moisturize the skin and ensures an even distribution of the essential oils, which is important in the case of babies and young children (see 'Babies, Infants and Children', pages 42–4). To avoid possible irritation always check the safety data (see pages 57–69) before using a new oil in the bath.

MASSAGE

Therapeutic massage is the main method used by professional aromatherapists, but it can be practised equally well at home – either on oneself, or on a friend or partner. If it is not possible to carry out a full body massage, then a foot massage using appropriate oils is an excellent alternative. When we massage the feet, we stimulate the rest of the body as well. This is because all the organs, glands and muscles in the human body have nerve endings located in the soles of the feet.

Aromatic oils can also be rubbed into particular areas of the body to help combat specific complaints: tense, aching shoulders should be kneaded using a soothing massage oil to relax the muscles; stomach ache or period pain can be eased with a gentle anti-spasmodic oil applied to the abdomen in a clockwise direction.

Massage can also be a very sensual experience, and between lovers can bring new depth to a relationship, as well as enhance sexual enjoyment. Some essential oils are renowned for their aphrodisiac effect!

For the purpose of massage, essential oils are mixed with a base oil or vegetable oil, such as sweet almond or grapeseed oil, before being applied to the body. The dilution should be in the region of 1–3 per cent, depending upon the type of oil used and the specific purpose. In general, complaints of a physical nature, such as aching muscles or rheumatism, require a stronger concentration than disorders related to the emotions, like depression or insomnia.

An easy way of calculating how much essential oil to add to a base oil is to measure the amount of base oil in millilitres and then add about half that number of drops of essential oil.

For example:

* to a 50ml bottle of base oil, add about 25 drops of essential oil – this gives a 2.5 per cent dilution. Add a few more drops for a physical remedy, a few less for the treatment of an emotional or psychological problem

* to 1 tablespoon (approximately 15ml) base oil add 6–9 drops of essential oil

* to 1 teaspoon (approximately 5ml) carrier oil add 2–3 drops of essential oil

VAPORIZED OILS

Vaporized oils can be used for a variety of reasons: a penetrating oil like *sweet basil*, for example, can scent a room and dispel unwanted odours; an antiseptic oil such as *eucalyptus* can rid a room of germs and help with respiratory complaints; and insecticides like *citronella* can be used to repel mosquitoes and other insects.

There are many vaporizing methods available. You can use an oil burner, or an electric diffuser, or simply add a few drops of oil to a bowl of hot water placed on a radiator. Avoid applying essential oils directly on to a light bulb, as this may cause the bulb to explode. If you wish to keep insects at bay, applying oil to hanging ribbons or to clothing can be very effective. A few drops of an expectorant essential oil such as *myrtle* put on to the pillow, on night clothes for the night, or on a hankie during the day, can help combat coughs and colds. These are all ways of ensuring that the vaporized oil will have an effect.

NEAT APPLICATION

In general, essential oils should not be applied neat to the skin due to their concentration. Some oils can cause irritation, a burning or tingling sensation when they are applied in an undiluted form. However, there are exceptions to this rule. *Lavender*, for example, can be applied directly to burns, insect bites, cuts or spots. Some essential oils can also be applied in minute amounts to the skin as perfumes – see below and page 54. But most oils should never be applied undiluted, unless specifically directed.

PERFUMES

Many essential oils are ideal as perfumes – either on their own or combined with others. *Ylang ylang* is renowned as a well-balanced fragrance in its own right and oils such as *rose, jasmine, neroli* and *sandalwood* are all very popular scents. Such oils can be dabbed on the wrist or behind the ears, either neat or diluted to 5 per cent in jojoba, coconut or a bland base oil (for example, 5 drops to 1 teaspoon of oil). Before using a new oil as a perfume always do a patch test first (see 'Safety Guidelines', page 20). Aromatic oils can also be used to scent hair, linen, clothes, paper, pot-pourris or other items. (See also pages 54–6.)

Pure essential oils have a totally different quality to synthetic perfumes because they are derived from natural sources. Artificially made perfumes do not have the subtle balance of constituents and the therapeutic qualities of real essential oils.

SKIN CARE

Skin and beauty care are central to the practice of aromatherapy. Receiving a full body massage in the hands of a professional aromatherapist is certainly a treat, but not essential for maintaining a clear and healthy complexion. Most of the aromatic recipes included in this book are simple to make, and regular treatment can be carried out at home.

Facial oils

These are made up in the same way as massage oils, except that the carrier oil as well as the essential oil can be adapted to the type of skin being treated. Additional carrier oils include avocado, olive, wheatgerm, hazelnut, apricot kernel, peach kernel, borage seed, carrot oil and evening primrose, as well as the more basic carrier oils which are sweet almond, grapeseed, jojoba and soya oil. (See 'Skin and Hair Care' on pages 44–50 for which oils to use for different skin types.)

A good basic recipe is 2 teaspoons of a basic carrier oil with 1 teaspoon of a specific carrier oil suited to skin type and 6–9 drops of essential oil.

Facial creams

An aromatic facial cream can be made by adding 8–10 drops of essential oil, according to skin type (see pages 45–50), to a commercial unscented cream (100g jar) or by making up a basic cream for oneself, such as Galen's Cold Cream:

10g beeswax

40g almond oil

40g rosewater

10 drops of *rose* essential oil

Shred the beeswax and put it into a Pyrex bowl together with the almond oil. Place the bowl in a pan of water over a gentle heat, and mix until the beeswax has melted. Warm the rosewater in the same fashion, and add to the wax and oil mixture bit by bit, beating all the time. Finally stir in the essential oil and put in the fridge to set.

This cream can be used for the face, the hands or for massage to the body. Other essential oils can be used in place of *rose*, according to skin type.

Gels

Water-based gels provide a useful non-oily medium for the application of essential oils, as an alternative to oils and creams. A gel can be used to dilute any essential oil for irritating skin conditions, such as eczema or athlete's foot, particularly if the skin is broken or sensitive. Vegetable oils are best avoided as a base if the skin is broken, since they prevent the skin forming a crust. This method is also suitable for general skin care, especially if the skin tends to be greasy. Add 2–3 drops of essential oil to a teaspoon of gel and mix well before applying to the skin.

Masks

Face masks have many benefits – they can nourish, rejuvenate, stimulate, cleanse or soothe the skin, and generally improve its texture and quality. Masks can be made from a wide range of natural ingredients including fruit, yoghurt, honey and clay. There are many different kinds of clay, but green clay is the most versatile, as it is a good antiseptic and is rich in minerals. An essential oil and clay mask is excellent for the treatment of acne and congested skin, for revitalizing dry complexions, for helping to balance combination skin as well as being generally rejuvenating.

A good basic recipe is 50g of green clay and 2 teaspoons of cornflower, mixed together and kept in a jar. When you want to make a mask, mix together 1 tablespoon of the basic mixture, 1 egg yolk, 1 teaspoon of water, and 3 drops of an essential oil suited to your skin type.

Flower waters

These are easy to make at home, and are beneficial for all types of skin. Simply add up to 30 drops of essential oil to a 100ml bottle of spring water, leave it to stand for up to a month, and then filter using coffee filter paper. *Lavender*, *rose* and *neroli* are the most traditional scents, but other oils such as *geranium* or *sandalwood* may also be used either individually or blended together.

A variety of essential oils can also be diluted in alcohol to make toilet waters, eau-de-colognes or after-shave lotions. For example, a traditional toilet water called Eau de Portugal can be made by mixing 20 drops of *sweet orange*, 5 drops of *bergamot*, 2 drops of *lemon*, 2 drops of *benzoin* and 1 drop of *geranium* in 1 tablespoon of vodka and 100ml of spring water. Shake well and leave it to mature for a month at least, then filter.

STEAM INHALATION

This method is especially suited to congested sinus, throat and chest infections. Add about 5 drops of an essential oil, such as *eucalyptus* or *peppermint*, to a bowl of steaming water, cover the head with a towel and breathe deeply for 3–10 minutes, keeping the eyes closed. Soaking in a steaming hot bath containing expectorant oils which are non-irritating to the skin, such as *pine needle* or *marjoram*, can also help clear congestion (see pages 28–9).

Steam inhalation also acts as a kind of facial 'sauna'. For example, the use of oils such as *tea tree* can help unblock the pores and clear the complexion of spots and blackheads.

COMPRESS

This is suited to a variety of first aid cases – use a hot compress for abscesses, muscular aches, pains and severe tension; a cold compress for bumps and bruises, headaches, migraines and sprains.

Prepare a hot compress by dipping a flannel or piece of cotton wool into a small bowl of steaming water to which has been added 3–5 drops of a soothing oil such as *lavender*, and then apply to the affected area. Make a cold compress by dipping a flannel or hankie in a bowl of cold water to which has been added 3–5 drops of a cooling oil such as *peppermint*, then wrap it round an ice cube before applying to the area concerned.

DOUCHE

This method can be very helpful in the treatment of urinary or genital conditions, such as pruritis (itching), cystitis or thrush (see pages

36 and 38.) The area can be bathed in a sitz bath or a bowl of water to which 3–5 drops of a suitable essence have been added – *cypress* and *lavender*, for example, can help to heal the perineum after childbirth. Alternatively, an enema pot or plastic douche can be bought from some chemists for vaginal disorders. Add 3–5 drops of a suitable essential oil to warm water and mix well before inserting – *bergamot* and *tea tree* may be used effectively for the treatment of thrush.

GARGLE

For the treatment of mouth ulcers, sore throats, bad breath or other mouth or gum infections (see page 30), simply add about 3 drops of an essential oil such as *fennel* to a glass of warm boiled water, mix well and gargle.

Safety Guidelines

In general, essential oils are safe to use in the home and experiencing and exploring their unique scents and individual properties is both helpful and inspiring. However, because of the high concentration and potency of the oils it is necessary to take some precautions into account, as you would with any other household item.

SAFETY DATA

Always check the specific safety data before using a new oil (see pages 57–69).

INTERNAL USE

Do not take essential oils internally. This rule is in accordance with the safety guidelines recommended by the International Federation of Aromatherapists. Essential oils do not mix with water, and in an undiluted form they may damage the delicate lining of the digestive tract. In addition, some essential oils are toxic if taken internally (see page 21).

NEAT APPLICATION

In general, essential oils should not be applied neat to the skin – always dilute them in a carrier oil or cream first. There are exceptions to this rule, such as the use of neat *lavender* for cuts, spots, burns, etc. Certain non-irritant essential oils, such as *ylang ylang* or *sandalwood*, may be applied neat to the skin as perfumes (check the safety data on pages 57–69). Always do a patch test first (see below), and keep well away from the eyes.

SKIN IRRITATION

Oils which may irritate the skin or cause an allergic reaction are *sweet basil, black pepper, cinnamon leaf, clove bud, eucalyptus, ginger, lemon, lemongrass, peppermint, pine needle* and *thyme*. These oils should be used in half the usual recommended dilutions and no more than 3 drops added to the bath. If irritation does occur, bathe the area with cold water.

SENSITIVE SKIN

Some oils, including *tea tree*, may cause skin irritation in people with very sensitive skins (see the safety data on pages 57–69). Since *tea tree* is such a useful oil (which may sometimes be used neat), it is important for those with sensitive skins to dilute it first in a non-oily cream or gel. Always do a patch test before using a new oil to check for individual sensitization.

PATCH TEST

Before applying any new oil to the skin, even as a perfume, always do a patch test. Simply put a few drops on the back of your wrist, cover with a plaster and leave for an hour or more. If irritation or redness occurs, bathe the area with cold water. For future use, reduce the concentration level by half or avoid the oil altogether.

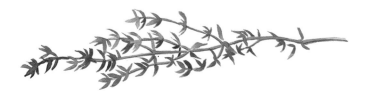

TOXICITY

Essential oils which should be used in moderation externally because of high toxicity levels are *aniseed, camphor, clove bud, eucalyptus, hyssop, nutmeg, oregano, sweet fennel* and *spanish sage.*

Hazardous oils such as *pennyroyal, mustard, sassafras, rue* and *mugwort* should not be used at all and are not included in this book.

PHOTOTOXICITY

Some oils are phototoxic, which means they cause skin pigmentation if exposed to direct sunlight. Do not use the following oils on the skin, either neat or in dilution, if the area will be exposed to the sun or ultra-violet light (as on a sunbed); *bergamot* (except bergapten-free oil, see page 57), *cumin, lemon, lime* or *orange.*

BABIES AND CHILDREN

Always dilute oils for babies and infants to at least half the recommended amount. For young children, avoid altogether the possibly toxic and irritant oils listed above. (See also 'Babies, Infants and Children', pages 42–4.)

Babies 0–12 months: use only 1 drop of *lavender, rose, roman/german chamomile, neroli* or *mandarin* essential oil, diluted in 1 teaspoon carrier oil for massage or bathing.

Infants 1–5 years: use only 2–3 drops of the 'safe' oils, i.e. those which are non-toxic and non-irritant, diluted in 1 teaspoon carrier oil for massage or bathing.

Children 6–12 years: use as for adults but in half the stated concentration.

Teenagers: use as directed for adults.

PREGNANCY

During pregnancy, use essential oils in half the usual stated amount because of the sensitivity of the growing foetus. Oils which are potentially

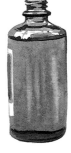

toxic or have emmenagogue properties (that is, they stimulate the uterus muscles) are contra-indicated.

The following oils should be avoided altogether: *basil, cinnamon leaf, citronella, clary sage, clove, hyssop, juniper, marjoram, myrrh, spanish sage, tarragon* and *thyme.*

The following oils are best avoided during the first four months of pregnancy: *atlas cedarwood, peppermint, rosemary* and *sweet fennel.* (See also 'Pregnancy and Childbirth', pages 39–41.)

HIGH BLOOD PRESSURE

Avoid the following oils in cases of this condition as they can raise the blood pressure: *hyssop, rosemary, sage* (all types) and *thyme.* (See also pages 34–5.)

EPILEPSY

Avoid the following oils in cases of epilepsy because they have a powerful effect on the nervous system: *sweet fennel, hyssop* and *sage* (all types).

ALCOHOL

The oil of *clary sage* should not be used in *any* form within a few hours of drinking alcohol. It can cause nausea and exaggerated drunkenness.

HOMEOPATHY

Homeopathic treatment is not compatible with the following oils due to their strength: *black pepper, camphor, eucalyptus* and *peppermint.*

STORAGE

Store in dark bottles, away from light and heat, and well out of the reach of children.

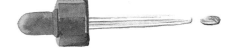

A GUIDE TO HOME USES

The Treatment of Common Complaints

FIRST AID

BRUISES AND BUMPS

❋ Minor bruises and bumps can be treated using a cold compress (such as a wet flannel or lint wrapped round an ice cube) to which has been added 3 drops of either *lavender, marjoram* or *geranium*.

❋ For quick pain relief, and to stop the swelling, apply neat *lavender*.

❋ If there is inflammation, 2 drops of *german chamomile* should be applied in 1 teaspoon of non-greasy cream or gel.

NOTE One of the most effective remedies for bruising is the homeopathic cream or tincture *Arnica*.

BURNS (MINOR) AND SUNBURN

❋ For minor household burns or scalds apply ice-cold water immediately for 10 minutes, then a couple of drops of neat *lavender*. Renew 3 times daily.

❋ Large areas of redness from sunburn can be soothed by adding 5–10 drops of *german chamomile* to a lukewarm bath and soaking for 10 minutes. More severe patches or blisters should be treated with a few drops of neat *lavender* oil.

❋ A good after-sun oil to treat dry, parched or red skin is to blend 2 drops each of *lavender, geranium* and *german chamomile* with 1 tablespoon almond oil (or moisturizing lotion) and massage in well after sunbathing.

CUTS, SORES AND SCARS

Essential oils are very useful for minor first aid since they can reduce the possibility of infection, encourage the skin to heal and help prevent scarring.

* Always clean a cut or sore carefully with a little cooled boiled water to which has been added 2 drops of any of the following antiseptic oils: *eucalyptus, lavender, lemon* or *tea tree*.

* For small cuts or grazes, apply 1–2 drops of neat *lavender* as needed. For larger injuries, add a few drops of *lavender* to a plaster or gauze to cover the wound. Renew the dressing 3 times daily.

* For infected cuts or splinters, apply 3 drops of *tea tree* or *german chamomile* diluted in 1 teaspoon of gel to the affected area 3 times daily, especially if there is inflammation.

* If the wound is bleeding, dab it with a gauze soaked in a bowl of cold water to which has been added 2 drops of *lemon*.

* If the cut or sore is weepy, a drop of the oil of *myrrh, benzoin* or *patchouli* may be applied to the dressing or used to bathe the wound, diluted in warm water.

* If a scar is slow to heal, make an ointment using 3 drops in total of either *neroli, rose, german chamomile, lavender* or *frankincense* (or a combination of these) in 1 teaspoon of wheatgerm oil (and, if possible, a little calendula and/or rosehip base oil). This should be applied regularly until the skin is healthy again.

INSECT BITES AND REPELLENTS

* To keep insects out of the house, use *citronella, lemongrass, thyme, peppermint, lavender, basil, eucalyptus, geranium* or *atlas cedarwood* essential oils in room vaporizers, plant sprays, or applied to hanging ribbons.

* Alternatively, an excellent blend can be made by mixing 2 drops each of *thyme, lavender* and *peppermint* with 8 drops of *lemongrass*. This can be used as an airborne deterrent blend in an oil burner, vaporizer or plant spray, or 6 drops may be added to 1 tablespoon of carrier oil or cream and applied directly to the skin.

* A simple method of keeping insects at bay, especially mosquitoes, is to rub a few drops of neat *lavender* on to exposed areas of the skin or on to clothing (it does not stain).

* Oils which keep moths away from linen include *lavender, patchouli, camphor, atlas cedarwood* and *basil.*

* When it comes to treating bites or stings, the most effective and simple remedy is neat *lavender* applied immediately to the sting and then re-applied at least 3 times a day. This works for mosquitoes, knats, bees, wasps and tics (as well as nettlerash). For tics, first apply a drop of neat *tea tree* to make them lose their grip, before removing.

* If there is a rash, swelling or inflammation, 3 drops of *german chamomile* should be applied in 1 teaspoon of non-greasy cream or gel.

MUSCULAR ACHES, PAINS AND SPRAINS

* Muscular pain as a result of over-exertion responds well to local massage. To ease aches and pains use 3 drops each of *lavender, rosemary* and *marjoram* in 1 tablespoon carrier oil, then rub well into the affected areas.

* Soaking in a hot bath is an easy and effective way of bringing instant relief. To aid relaxation and ease pain, add 5–10 drops of either *lavender, marjoram, clary sage* or *german/roman chamomile* to the water, or use a combination of these.

* To relieve muscle spasm or if a particular spot is very tight, apply a hot compress, to which has been added a couple of drops of *marjoram,* to the area. Alternatively, mix 1 drop each of *black pepper, marjoram* and *rosemary* in 1 teaspoon carrier oil and massage deeply on and around the area.

* To help prepare the muscles for action and increase muscle tone use 3 drops each of *rosemary* and *juniper* with 2 drops of *black pepper* in 1 tablespoon carrier oil for local massage; or add 5–10 drops of *rosemary, grapefruit* or *juniper* to the bath.

* To treat a sprain, prepare a cold compress to which has been added a few drops of either *lavender* or *roman/german chamomile* (or both), apply to the injury and repeat as often as possible to reduce the swelling. Do not massage. Wrap in a bandage and rest the joint as much as possible.

25

RHEUMATISM, ARTHRITIS AND BURSITIS

Rheumatism is a general word for pain and inflammation affecting the joints and surrounding muscles, and includes arthritis and bursitis.

Bursitis is one of the most common rheumatic conditions, usually affecting the shoulders, elbows (tennis elbow) and knees (housemaid's knee). There are several kinds of arthritis, with various different causes, but all types signify a friction between the bones of a joint resulting in pain, loss of mobility, possible inflammation and eventual deformity.

Conflict on an inner or emotional level often contributes to the development of this disease, as does a poor diet which can lead to a build up of toxins in the body, with uric acid being deposited as crystals in the joint spaces. Climate is also an important consideration, and damp is often an aggravating factor.

✻ Use a detoxifying massage oil blend at least once a week to improve circulation and eliminate toxins from the body: 1 tablespoon carrier oil with 9 drops in total of *juniper, cypress, pine needle, fennel* or *lemon* (or a combination of these). If it is not possible to have a full body massage, then gentle self-massage to the affected areas is of great benefit.

✻ Bathing also helps to eliminate toxins and ease pain: use 5–10 drops of *fennel, juniper* or *pine needle* (or a combination of these) in a morning bath; 5–10 drops of *lavender, clary sage* or *roman/german chamomile* (or a combination of these) in an evening bath.

✻ A hot compress using a couple of drops of *rosemary, black pepper, lavender* or *marjoram* (or a combination of these) helps to ease local pain; a strong rub using 1 teaspoon carrier oil with 1 drop each of the above oils is also helpful.

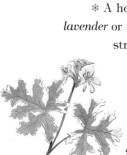

✻ For bursitis, mix 3 drops each of *rosemary, geranium* and *eucalyptus* with 1 tablespoon carrier oil, and rub gently into the area.

✻ A good anti-rheumatic oil for general application is 2 drops each of *lemon, rosemary, pine needle* and *juniper* with 1 drop of *ginger* and *black pepper* in 1 tablespoon of carrier oil.

INFECTIOUS AND RESPIRATORY ILLNESSES

ASTHMA AND HAYFEVER

Asthma, characterized by attacks of wheezing and shortness of breath, is very often an allergy-induced disorder, starting in childhood and frequently going hand in hand with bronchitis, hayfever and other allergic reactions such as eczema. An attack can be triggered by an infection like a cold or by allergens such as pollen or dust, but is largely related to over-exertion and stress, especially in those of a nervous disposition.

Hayfever is due to an allergic reaction to pollen or other irritants, and since some essential oils can induce allergic reactions, extreme care must be taken in the choice of a suitable remedy. The following combinations can help to alleviate the problem, but because asthma and hayfever affect people in different ways, the treatment is often a case of trial and error.

✳ The most useful oil for hayfever and asthma is *peppermint*, since it is anti-spasmodic (soothing), expectorant and helps to clear the head. Use regularly in the bath (3 drops only), in a vaporizer or on the pillow.

✳ Other soothing oils, such as *bergamot, roman/german chamomile, clary sage, frankincense, lavender, neroli* and *rose*, can all help to ease nervous tension or anxiety: add 5–10 drops to the bath water.

✳ Regular massage using a relaxing, soothing blend can help prevent tension and anxiety building up. A recommended mixture is 2 drops each of *roman/german chamomile, bergamot* and *lavender* in 1 tablespoon carrier oil.

✳ During an attack, asthma and hayfever sufferers can put the following oils on a tissue to inhale: 3 drops in total of *roman/german chamomile, peppermint* or *lavender* (or a combination of these).

✳ For everyday use, add a few drops of *frankincense, roman/german chamomile, lavender* or *atlas cedarwood* to a vaporizer to create a relaxing atmosphere in the home.

COMMON COLDS AND SINUSITIS

❋ The two most useful oils for stimulating the immune system and fighting the cold virus are *eucalyptus* and *tea tree*. At the first sign of a cold appearing, use these oils in a vaporizer or apply a few drops to the pillow or a tissue for inhalation throughout the day and night.

❋ For shivers, headaches and aching muscles take a warm bath with 3–5 drops each of *lavender* and *marjoram*. This will also encourage restful sleep.

❋ *Eucalyptus, tea tree, thyme, peppermint* and *bergamot* help to reduce temperature and fight infection. A few drops of these oils can be used in a vaporizer or added to a dish of steaming water placed on a radiator in the sick room.

❋ The best way to combat congestion, sinusitis and catarrh is to use steam inhalations. Add a few drops of *rosemary, peppermint* or *eucalyptus* to a bowl of hot water and inhale deeply for 3–10 minutes, keeping the eyes closed. In addition, use the above oils in a vaporizer or add a few drops to a tissue for inhalation throughout the day.

❋ To further clear the head of stuffiness and help fight viral infection add 3 drops each of *rosemary, ginger* and *lavender,* OR *spanish sage, cardomon* and *pine needle* to a steaming bath.

❋ For a sore throat, add 3 drops in total of *clary sage, spanish sage, tea tree* or *geranium* (or a combination of these) to a glass of warm boiled water with a little fresh lemon juice (an excellent antiseptic). Mix well and gargle. (Not to be used by children under five.)

COUGHS AND BRONCHITIS

Coughs can be dry and irritating or they can be accompanied by mucus discharge, especially in association with a cold or with bronchitis.

Bronchitis indicates an inflammation of the bronchial tubes, accompanied by coughing and an over-production of mucus. Acute bronchitis usually starts with a cold or sore throat, which then develops into a fever that lasts a few days. Chronic bronchitis is a long-term condition, without fever, which is aggravated by smoking, a damp climate, air pollution and poor nutrition (especially too many dairy products).

✳ When there is fever present, *eucalyptus*, *tea tree*, *thyme*, *peppermint* and *bergamot* help to reduce temperature and fight infection. A few drops of these oils can be used in a vaporizer or added to a dish of steaming water placed on a radiator in the sick room.

✳ The best way to combat excess mucus, congestion and catarrh is to use steam inhalations. Add a few drops of *rosemary*, *peppermint* or *eucalyptus* (or a combination of these) to a bowl of hot water and inhale deeply for 3–10 minutes, keeping the eyes closed. In addition, add a few drops to a tissue for inhalation throughout the day.

✳ There are many essential oils with balsamic properties which are soothing and help to loosen mucus (for dry or irritating coughs), the most effective being *atlas cedarwood*, *benzoin*, *myrrh*, *frankincense*, *sandalwood* and *pine needle*. A few drops of any of these oils can be used in a vaporizer or added to the bath water.

✳ A local back and chest massage oil, which is effective against bronchitis, coughs and catarrh, can be made by blending 2 drops each of *eucalyptus*, *thyme*, *benzoin* and *ginger* with 1 tablespoon carrier oil. Alternatively, for a dry cough simply add 3 drops of *pine needle*, *sandalwood* or *atlas cedarwood* (or a combination of these) to 1 tablespoon of base oil.

✳ A useful oil for night coughs in children and adults is *myrtle*, since it helps to fight infection but is not too stimulating, which might otherwise prevent sleep. Use a few drops on the pillow or on night clothes or in a vaporizer.

FEVER AND INFECTION

Although essential oils can help provide relief during an infectious illness, as well as reduce its duration and prevent it from spreading, in cases of high fever, severe infection or an acute childhood illness, the following home treatments should never be used as a substitute for professional help.

❋ The two most useful oils for stimulating the immune system and fighting viruses of all kinds, including flu, are *eucalyptus* and *tea tree*. Use these oils in a vaporizer in the sick room or put a few drops on the pillow or on a hankie for use throughout the day and night.

❋ For shivers, headaches and aching muscles take a warm bath with 4 drops each of *lavender* and *marjoram*. This will also encourage restful sleep. *Roman/german chamomile* is helpful in overcoming anxiety or insomnia.

❋ When there is fever present, *eucalyptus*, *tea tree*, *thyme*, *peppermint* and *bergamot* help to reduce temperature and fight infection. A few drops of these oils can be used in a vaporizer or added to a dish of steaming water placed on a radiator in the sick room.

❋ For a sore throat, add 2 drops in total of *clary sage*, *spanish sage*, *tea tree* or *geranium* (and a little fresh lemon juice) to a glass of warm boiled water, mix well and gargle. (Not to be used by children under five.)

MOUTH, TOOTH AND GUM INFECTIONS

❋ A traditional remedy for toothache is to put 1 drop of *clove* oil on to a cotton bud and apply to the tooth. (Do not swallow.)

❋ Disease of the gums (gingivitis) is a common cause of tooth loss, and care of the gums is vital to health. A good mouth rinse to prevent bleeding or swollen gums is 3 drops in total of *clove*, *fennel*, *clary sage*, *spanish sage* or *thyme* (or a combination of these) in a cup of warm boiled water together with a pinch of sea salt. If the infection is severe, a few drops of neat *myrrh* should be massaged on to the affected area.

❋ To treat mouth ulcers, dry the affected area and dab twice daily with *bergamot* (so long as it is bergapten-free, see page 57), *tea tree* or *myrrh*. In addition, rinse the mouth out using 4 drops of *bergamot*, *tea tree* or *myrrh* in a glass of warm boiled water.

❋ For swelling and pain resulting from infected gums or wisdom teeth, mix 3 drops in total of *lavender* or *roman/german chamomile* (or a combination of both) in 1 teaspoon carrier oil, and massage into the cheeks. A hot compress also helps ease pain.

＊ A good remedy for bad breath or halitosis is to use the following mixture regularly: 100ml of cheap brandy or vodka, 10 drops each of *thyme* and *peppermint* with 5 drops each of *myrrh* and *fennel*. To use, mix 2 or 3 teaspoons in half a cup of warm water, and rinse the mouth out twice daily.

STRESS-RELATED CONDITIONS

Stress is *the* modern-day disease, and one we all suffer from at some time or another. When we are stressed we become less resistant to all kinds of illness that affect the body, the emotions and the mind. Allowing space for ourselves is something that many of us find difficult, whether because of work or through family pressures.

The use of aromatics can help to lift anxiety and bring about a change in our state of mind. This is one of the most traditional uses of essential oils, and the reason they have played an important role in both religious and secular rituals for thousands of years.

With the present-day emphasis on materialism and the achievement of external goals, it is important to keep in touch with ourselves on an inner level, and the use of aromatics can help to facilitate this. Engaging in the ritual of a candlelit aromatic bath, or burning essences to create a relaxed atmosphere in a room, or using essential oils for massage or to aid meditation, are all ways of slowing down the mind and of becoming more attuned to the moment. It is also important, of course, to try to deal with the causes of stress directly, and if necessary to seek professional help.

Because of the emotional elements which are at play in stress-related conditions, the choice of essential oils depends largely on the causes of the problem, and the temperament of each individual and how they respond under pressure. The following aromatic recipes may provide a few ideas.

DEPRESSION AND ANXIETY

Depression can take many forms, and it is important to try to understand the causes and deal with them directly. Essential

31

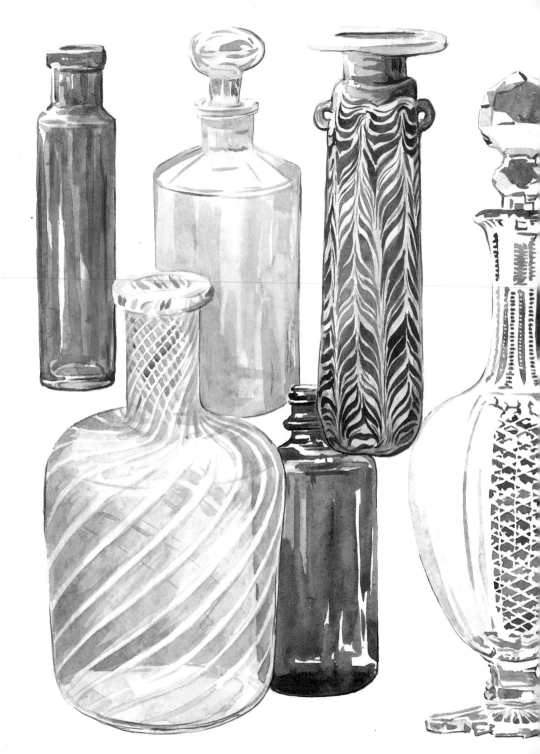

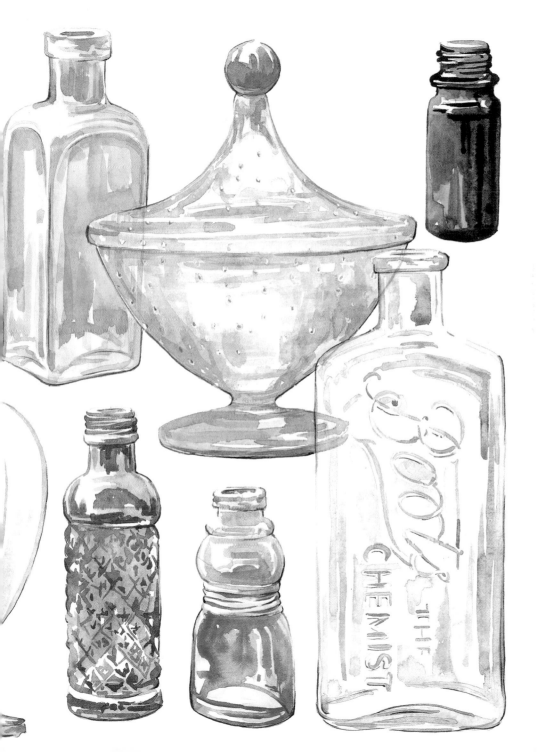

oils can help alleviate the symptoms, but since this is primarily an emotional complaint, the method of treatment is very much an individual matter.

✳ If the depression is associated with lethargy and lack of energy, oils such as *sweet basil, bergamot, geranium, neroli, jasmine* and *rose* can be uplifting and energizing, used in the bath, in a vaporizer, or as perfumes. Practising massage either on oneself or with a friend can be of great benefit, combining both the comforting effect of touch and the remedial effect of the oils.

✳ If the depression is associated with restlessness and anxiety, then the more sedating and soothing oils such as *chamomile, clary sage, lavender, atlas cedarwood, marjoram, vetiver, ylang ylang* and *sandalwood* can help encourage a relaxed state of mind. Aromatic bathing, massage, scenting the home and using these oils as perfumes, are all ways of bringing enjoyment and pleasure both to the individual and to those around them.

✳ Those oils which have traditionally been used as incenses, such as *benzoin, atlas cedarwood, cypress, frankincense, juniper* and *sandalwood*, can help bring about a calm state of mind, used either as perfumes or in a vaporizer. Since there are so many oils to choose from when it comes to helping depression, one of the best ways of deciding is simply to select the scent which appeals and gives pleasure in that moment.

DIGESTIVE UPSETS

Digestive upsets are often the result of anxiety or stress. They respond well to the external application of essential oils, but this is often enhanced by the use of herbal remedies, such as peppermint, chamomile or fennel tea.

✳ Stomach ache of nervous origin can be helped by gentle massage to the abdomen in a clockwise direction using 9 drops in total of *roman/german chamomile, lavender* or *marjoram* (or a combination of these) in 1 tablespoon carrier oil. *Neroli* is also especially soothing in cases of nerves or emotional upsets, used in the bath, in a vaporizer or as a massage oil.

✳ For indigestion with wind, use 9 drops in total of *fennel* or *peppermint* (or a combination of both) in 1 tablespoon carrier oil for massage as indicated above.

 ✳ To help ease constipation, use 9 drops in total of *rosemary, lemon* or *peppermint* (or a combination of these) in 1 tablespoon carrier oil for massage as indicated above.

 ✳ If there is diarrhoea or a viral infection is suspected, use 9 drops in total of *eucalyptus, tea tree* or *thyme* (or a combination of these) in 1 tablespoon carrier oil for massage as indicated above. A warm bath with 4 drops of *geranium* and 2 drops of *ginger* is also recommended.

 ✳ The other spice oils are also very beneficial to help relieve pain and promote digestion, used in minute amounts in massage oils or baths. They include *black pepper, carrot seed, clove, cardomon, cinnamon, coriander* and *ginger.*

FATIGUE, POOR CIRCULATION AND LOW BLOOD PRESSURE (HYPOTENSION)

Fatigue can be caused by exhaustion and stress, or can be related to feelings of lethargy due to a slow metabolic rate. Poor circulation and low blood pressure often occur together, and in both cases stimulating essences are advised. Attention to diet and exercise is also very beneficial, especially for those with a sedentary lifestyle.

 ✳ *Rosemary* is the most useful oil for this condition, being stimulating and a tonic. Use 5–10 drops of *cypress* or *rosemary*, OR 3–5 drops of *peppermint, sweet basil* or *spanish sage* in the bath.

 ✳ A vigorous massage using 7 drops of *rosemary* and 2 drops of *black pepper* in 1 tablespoon carrier oil also helps to stimulate the system.

 ✳ Exhaustion and fatigue of a more emotional nature can be helped by mentally reviving and uplifting oils such as *jasmine, rose, bergamot* or *geranium,* used in vaporizers or as perfumes.

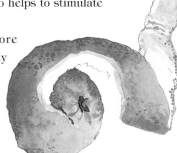

33

✳ Excessive fatigue can be counteracted with refreshing and uplifting bath oils which may be used in the morning or before going out in the evening after a heavy day. Recommended bath blends are 3–5 drops each of *rosemary* and *bergamot*, OR *rosemary* and *petitgrain*, OR *geranium* and *sweet basil*.

HEADACHES AND MIGRAINE

✳ For tension headaches apply neat *lavender* to the temples or to the back of the neck; to ease strain and tension, massage the shoulders and neck using 1 teaspoon carrier oil with 3 drops in total of *lavender* or *marjoram* (or a combination of both).

✳ For congested headaches due to blocked sinuses, use a few drops of *peppermint* or *eucalyptus* on a tissue to inhale throughout the day, in a vaporizer or added to a bowl of steaming water as an inhalation.

✳ Migraine is most commonly a food-related complaint, but an attack can also be triggered by an increase in stress or anxiety. A cold compress placed on the temples using 1 drop of *lavender* can help to ease discomfort during an attack. As a preventative measure, soothing and relaxing oils such as *lavender, roman/german chamomile, marjoram, neroli* and *sandalwood* should be used on a daily basis in baths, massages, vaporizers or as perfumes.

HIGH BLOOD PRESSURE (HYPERTENSION)

Although aromatherapy treatments have been found to reduce blood pressure significantly, it is vital also to review issues such as diet, exercise and general lifestyle. In addition, garlic, either eaten raw or taken as perles or tablets, has been found to help control high blood pressure. Stimulants, such as tea, coffee and alcohol, should be reduced or eliminated.

✳ Regular massage is particularly helpful for this condition and can dramatically reduce high blood pressure – an excellent blend for massage at home is 3 drops each of *ylang ylang, lavender* and *marjoram* (or used individually) in 1 tablespoon carrier oil.

✻ The use of other relaxing and sedative oils such as *bergamot, roman/german chamomile, frankincense* or *sandalwood* is also effective. Use 5–10 drops of any of these oils (or a combination of them) in the bath, in a vaporizer or as a perfume.

✻ 5–10 drops of any of the cleansing and detoxifying oils, which include *fennel, lemon, grapefruit* and *juniper*, are also beneficial when used in the bath (or for massage).

NERVOUS TENSION AND INSOMNIA

✻ For the workaholic, some good soothing bath combinations to use before retiring are 3–5 drops each of *lavender* and *marjoram*, OR *roman/german chamomile* and *neroli*, OR *lavender* and *frankincense*. Other oils which are also very beneficial for relaxation are *vetiver, sandalwood, clary sage, ylang ylang* and *atlas cedarwood*.

✻ Emotional stress and nervous tension expresses itself in different ways – some people cope by becoming over-active, some people become depressed, while others collapse. Some good basic bath combinations which are supportive and comforting are 3–5 drops each of *bergamot* and *clary sage* (anti-depressant), OR *sandalwood* and *rose* (soothing), OR *jasmine* and *geranium* (gently stimulating).

✻ A full body massage at the hands of a qualified aromatherapist can do much to alleviate stress, but massage can also be carried out in the home. A recommended blend for general tension/irritability is 2 drops each of *lavender, ylang ylang* and *clary sage* in 1 tablespoon carrier oil.

✻ Tension is often held in the body, especially in the neck and shoulder areas. A good massage blend for easing muscular tension and general aches and pains is 3 drops of *marjoram, lavender* or *roman/german chamomile* (or a combination of these) in 1 teaspoon sweet almond oil.

✻ The best oils for the insomnia that often accompanies stress are *lavender, marjoram, vetiver, roman/german chamomile* and *neroli*. Use in the bath, or put a few drops on the pillow or in a vaporizer in the bedroom before retiring. Herbal remedies, such as hop, valarian or skullcap tea, are also useful.

Women, Pregnancy and Children

WOMEN'S HEALTH

CELLULITIS

Although aromatherapy is very successful in helping to combat cellulite, this obviously needs to be backed up by exercise, dietary measures and, if possible, professional lymphatic massage (which encourages elimination of toxins via the lymphatic system). Hormonal imbalance, as well as stress and too much tea, coffee and alcohol, which all increase toxicity levels, also contribute to this condition.

 ✳ These stimulating, toxin-eliminating bath oil blends should be used on successive days: 3–4 drops each of *rosemary* and *juniper*, OR *lemon* and *grapefruit*, OR *fennel* and *geranium*. They can alternatively be applied to a loofah or massage glove and rubbed into the affected areas while bathing. Experiment with your own combinations of the above oils.

 ✳ A good detoxifying massage oil can be made by blending 2 drops each of *rosemary, geranium* and *juniper* and 1 drop of *black pepper* with 1 tablespoon of a carrier oil.

 ✳ General massage also helps to improve the circulation as well as reduce cellulite. Oils such as *carrot seed, cypress, thyme, spanish sage, rosemary* and *mandarin* are also of benefit here.

CYSTITIS AND PRURITIS (ITCHING)

Cystitis, which is an infection of the bladder, is characterized by a painful burning sensation while passing water. Pruritis, or itching, is an irritating condition which often accompanies a mild vaginal infection. Take garlic perles, drink plenty of water and keep tea, coffee, alcohol and spices to a minimum. Avoid tight-fitting clothes and nylon underwear.

 ✳ For cystitis, make up a solution (well shaken) using 5 drops each of *roman/german chamomile* and *bergamot* in 1 pint of cooled boiled water. Using a piece of soaked cotton wool, swab the opening of the urethra frequently (if possible, each time after passing water).

* In addition make up a massage oil using 3 drops each of *roman/german chamomile*, *bergamot* and *lavender* with 1 tablespoon carrier oil. This blend should be massaged into the lower back and abdomen twice daily.

* To help combat cystitis and pruritis, it is beneficial to bathe frequently using bactericidal essential oils. Add 5–10 drops of either *lavender*, *roman/german chamomile*, *juniper*, *sandalwood*, *tea tree* or *bergamot* to a warm bath, or add 2–3 drops to a bidet for local washing.

MENSTRUAL PROBLEMS

Essential oils can help to combat menstrual disorders on a variety of levels, because they are able to operate on the emotional and the physical sides simultaneously.

* For period pains, gently massage the abdomen and lower back with the following blend: 9 drops of *lavender*, *clary sage* or *marjoram* (or a combination of these) to 1 tablespoon carrier oil. Alternatively, add a few drops of *clary sage* to a hot compress (or use a hankie wrapped round a hot water bottle), and apply to the abdomen. (Remember, *clary sage* should not be used within a few hours of drinking alcohol.)

* The effects of pre menstrual tension can be eased by taking regular baths which help to relieve tension. Add 5–10 drops of either *lavender*, *clary sage*, *neroli* or *rose* to the bath water. In addition, 500mg of evening primrose oil should be taken daily in the week before the period.

* To help regulate heavy flow, make a massage oil blend using 9 drops of *cypress*, *geranium* or *rose* (or a combination of these) in 1 tablespoon carrier oil to rub on the abdomen. In addition use 5–10 drops of any of the above oils in the bath. Diet, exercise and emotional factors should also be assessed.

* To help promote or normalize scanty menstruation, make a massage oil blend using 9 drops of *clary sage*, *myrrh* or *roman chamomile* (or a

37

combination of these) in 1 tablespoon carrier oil to rub on the abdomen. In addition, use 5–10 drops of any of the above oils in the bath. Diet (poor diet, anaemia and being run down often accompany this problem), exercise and emotional factors should also be assessed.

OEDEMA (WATER RETENTION)

Although this is not an exclusively female complaint, oedema often occurs during the latter stages of pregnancy. It may also be caused by being overweight or other factors such as food allergies, standing for long periods or hormonal imbalance. It most commonly occurs in the ankles, but can also be found in the hands, stomach, or around the eyes.

 ✻ The most useful oils are *fennel, geranium* and *rosemary*. Add 9 drops of any one (or a combination of these) to 1 tablespoon carrier oil or cream and massage gently at the site of the swelling. Legs should be massaged with upward strokes.

 ✻ Alternatively, massage the soles of the feet with 2–3 drops of *cypress* in 1 teaspoon carrier oil.

 ✻ For swollen ankles, submerge in a lukewarm footbath containing a few drops of *cypress, fennel, geranium* or *rosemary*.

 ✻ Take warm baths containing 5–10 drops of any of the following oils: *lemon, mandarin, orange, fennel, grapefruit, rosemary, geranium* or *petitgrain*.

 ✻ Swelling and puffiness can also be relieved by applying a cold compress using 1 teaspoon witch hazel lotion (available from chemists) with 2 drops of *roman/german chamomile* to the affected area.

THRUSH (CANDIDA) AND LEUCORRHOEA

Thrush is a form of fungal infection, which affects warm, moist parts of the body, but most commonly occurs in the vagina, where symptoms include itching and a thick milky discharge.

Leucorrhoea is an inflammation of the vagina caused by the proliferation of unwanted bacteria or fungi, resulting in a thick white or yellow discharge.

Both conditions are aggravated by tight clothing, nylon underwear, harsh bubble baths, and the use of antibiotics. Most cases of thrush and leucorrhoea respond well to the use of *tea tree* oil.

❋ Add 5–10 drops of *tea tree* to the bath water daily (check sensitivity first) or a few drops to a sitz bath for a local wash.

❋ Make a douche by mixing 10 drops of *tea tree* with 1 pint of cooled boiled water and bathe the area using an enema pot, or soak a tampon in the above solution and insert into the vagina.

❋ Other oils of benefit which may be used in the bath include *geranium, juniper, lavender, rose* and *bergamot*: add 5–10 drops to the bath water.

PREGNANCY AND CHILDBIRTH

PREPARING FOR MOTHERHOOD

More and more women wish to deliver their baby in as natural and as active a way possible, without the use of drugs. There are now many books available on the subject, which cover issues such as nutrition, exercise or herbal remedies (for example, raspberry tea), all of which can help to make pregnancy and the birth easier and more enjoyable. Essential oils are being used increasingly by nurses and midwives in this context.

Using essential oils during pregnancy and to help with childbirth can be very beneficial in a variety of ways, but there are some precautions to be taken, due to the sensitivity of the womb and the unborn foetus.

1. Use all essential oils at half the usual stated amount during pregnancy.

2. The oils which should be avoided altogether are *basil, cinnamon leaf, citronella, clary sage, clove, hyssop, juniper, marjoram, myrrh, spanish sage, tarragon* and *thyme*.

3. The oils which are best avoided during the first four months of pregnancy are *atlas cedarwood, fennel, peppermint* and *rosemary*.

PREGNANCY

✳ An excellent oil to help prevent stretch marks can be made by blending 2 drops of *lavender* and 1 drop each of *neroli* and *frankincense* with 1 tablespoon wheatgerm oil – for light massage daily to the belly and breasts. This oil can also help to get rid of existing stretch marks.

✳ In addition wheatgerm oil can also be rubbed into the perineum to help prepare for the birth. Research has shown that massaging the perineum for 5–10 minutes daily in the last six weeks of pregnancy can help prevent tearing.

✳ Aromatic bathing offers great pleasure and relief, especially towards the end of pregnancy. Add 3–5 drops of any of the following oils to the bath: uplifting oils like *bergamot, orange, mandarin, geranium* and *jasmine* or relaxing oils like *sandalwood, rose, patchouli, ylang ylang, frankincense, chamomile* and *lavender.*

✳ Pamper yourself during pregnancy – use the following essential oils as perfumes or as soothing air fresheners to overcome anxiety and encourage a relaxed attitude to the forthcoming birth: *lavender* to relax, *roman/german chamomile* to calm the mind, *bergamot* and *mandarin* to uplift, *rose* or *jasmine* to comfort.

✳ Gentle massage can be very enjoyable during pregnancy, and can help with a wide variety of problems, such a back pain. To soothe back pain and relax the body, lie on one side and ask a friend or partner to use the following blend, applied to the lower back: 3 drops each of *lavender* and *roman/german chamomile* in 1 tablespoon of base oil or cream.

✳ Oedema, fatigue, varicose veins, constipation and other digestive problems are also common (see their entries). Always take care to avoid contra-indicated oils, and use in low dilutions only.

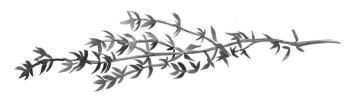

LABOUR

＊ A traditional and useful massage oil to help prepare for the birth and strengthen the uterus muscles is to blend 2 drops of *jasmine* with 1 drop of *nutmeg* in 1 teaspoon of carrier oil. Rub the oil on to the lower abdomen each day, for two weeks prior to the expected delivery.

＊ During the birth, and in preparing to bring the baby into the home, the use of vaporized oils to scent the environment can create an uplifting, relaxed mood. They also prevent the spread of airborne bacteria. Use a few drops of *lavender, frankincense* or *bergamot* in a vaporizer, or in a bowl of hot water on a radiator.

＊ Pain relief during labour can be aided by firm massage to the lower back using the following blend: 5 drops of *clary sage*, 2 drops each of *rose* and *lavender* in 1 tablespoon carrier oil.

AFTER THE DELIVERY

＊ To help heal the perineum after the birth, add 2 drops of *cypress* and 3 drops of *lavender* to a shallow bath, and soak. Repeat each day. This also helps to prevent infection.

＊ It is common to feel many mixed emotions after the birth. Post-natal depression can be helped by the use of uplifting and comforting oils, such as *lavender, bergamot, jasmine, rose* and *neroli. Geranium* can help to normalize hormonal imbalance and regulate mood swings. Use in the bath, for massage or in vaporizers.

＊ Engorged breasts can be soothed using a cold compress, or through gentle massage using 2–3 drops of *peppermint* oil to 1 tablespoon base oil or cream.

＊ For sore nipples, blend 1 drop of *rose, benzoin* or *lavender* in 1 teaspoon of non-oily cream or gel between feeds. Wipe off using a bland cream before each feed.

NOTE Calendula or chamomile ointment are also useful soothing remedies for cracked nipples.

BABIES, INFANTS AND CHILDREN

BABIES AND INFANTS

Babies and infants respond especially well to natural healing methods, but their extra sensitivity must be taken into account. Do not attempt to substitute a home remedy for professional treatment if it is needed.

    * **Babies 0–12 months:** use only 1 drop of either *lavender, rose, roman/german chamomile, neroli* or *mandarin* essential oil, diluted in 1 teaspoon carrier oil for massage or bathing.

    * **Infants 1–5 years:** use only 2–3 drops of the 'safe' essential oils diluted in 1 teaspoon carrier oil for massage or bathing, that is avoid all those oils which are potentially toxic or which may cause skin irritation. See 'Safety Guidelines' on pages 19–22 for which oils to avoid.

OLDER CHILDREN

Older children enjoy the stimulation of different scents. By the age of six they can recognize a wide range of smells, and enjoy being introduced to new experiences. It is fun to choose an oil to put in the bath or use as a scent. *Orange, mandarin* and *lavender* are popular with children because they are familiar and sweet. Add about 5 drops to the bath at bedtime.

    * **Children 6–12 years:** use as for adults but in half the stated concentration.

    * **Teenagers:** use as directed for adults.

COMMON CHILDHOOD COMPLAINTS

Many common childhood complaints can be treated with essential oils. Always check the dilution with the guidelines above.

    * Nappy rash in babies and infants can be prevented by regular bathing using 1 drop of either *lavender* or *roman/german chamomile* diluted in 1 teaspoon carrier oil. If nappy rash does occur add 1 drop of *tea tree* or *roman/german chamomile* to 1 teaspoon of a non-greasy baby cream

and apply gently at each nappy change. Nappy rash is often caused by thrush, see page 38.

❋ Restlessness and insomnia in babies, infants and older children can be helped by the use of *lavender, rose, roman/german chamomile* or *neroli* in the bath or for massage. Alternatively, use a vaporizer in the bedroom (ensure it is out of reach), or put a drop or two of oil on the pillow or on the pyjamas or nightie.

❋ Tummy ache and colic in babies, infants and older children can be eased by mixing 1–3 drops of *lavender* or *roman chamomile* in 1 teaspoon carrier oil, and gently massaging the lower back or stomach in a clockwise direction.

❋ Teething pain in babies and infants can be relieved by mixing 1 drop of *roman/german chamomile* in 1 teaspoon of carrier oil and massaging into the cheek.

❋ For cuts, spots, insect bites and other skin blemishes for infants over one year old, apply 1 drop of neat *lavender*.

❋ See also pages 23–35 for other common complaints.

INFECTIOUS ILLNESSES

The most useful oil for stimulating the immune system and fighting viruses of all kinds in children, including flu, chickenpox and measles, is *tea tree*. A few drops should be used in a vaporizer or put on the pillow or on a hankie for use throughout the day and night.

❋ For fever and whooping cough add a few drops of *bergamot* to a vaporizer or in a dish of steaming water placed on a radiator in the sick room. Steam vaporizations are especially useful during whooping cough to help relieve the coughing.

❋ Colds and coughs in infants and older children respond well to the use of essential oils. Put a drop or two of *myrtle, marjoram, atlas cedarwood* or *tea tree* on the pillow or on the pyjamas or nightie. Alternatively, use a few drops of any of the above oils in a vaporizer in the bedroom (ensure it is well out of reach).

* For infants and children add 2–4 drops of *orange* or *mandarin* to the bath at the first signs of a cold developing.

* To help reduce itching and prevent scarring from chickenpox, make a lotion using 50ml witch hazel, 50ml rosewater, with 2 drops each of *german chamomile, tea tree* and *lavender* and dab on to the blisters. Alternatively, and especially if the child is under five, add up to 3 drops of *lavender* or *german chamomile* to a warm bath with a handful of colloidal oatmeal (available from some chemists) and soak for 10 minutes at least twice a day.

B e a u t y , P e r f u m e s   a n d   P l e a s u r e

SKIN AND HAIR CARE

Essential oils are ideally suited to skin care, for they are readily absorbed and have the ability to penetrate through to the underlying layers of the skin, which are alive and active, unlike the outer dead layer of cells that are constantly being shed. Essential oils stimulate cellular regeneration, improve the circulation and help to eliminate toxins at a fundamental level. Skin that has been treated with aromatic oils thus becomes more dynamic and healthy. In addition, because the oils are able to travel in the bloodstream and lymphatic system, skin treatments using essential oils are vitalizing to the body as a whole.

The natural acid/alkaline balance of healthy skin has a PH value of 4.8–6. When a substance has a PH value of less than 7 it is acidic; when it is more than 7 it is alkaline. Most synthetic detergents and soaps are alkaline and can upset the natural acid mantle that protects against germs, dirt and invasive bacteria. It is therefore important that you do not strip the skin of this protective mantle and only use substances like essential oils which have a neutral PH value (between 6.5–7).

＊ Adding to the bath 5–10 drops of a suitable essence (according to skin type) is a convenient way of treating the entire body.

ACNE AND SPOTS

This common skin complaint is caused by over-activity of the sebaceous glands, and is most common during adolescence, the menopause and at times of hormonal imbalance or change, such as before menstruation. Poor diet, lack of exercise, stress and anxiety can further aggravate the condition.

＊ Apply an aromatic flower water as a toner/cleanser to the skin morning and evening. To prepare, mix 25ml witch hazel, 75ml rosewater with 5 drops each of *bergamot, geranium* and *lavender*. Let it mature for up to a month, then filter before use with coffee filter paper. (It is a good idea to prepare a whole batch in one go.)

＊ Use a light facial oil containing 2 teaspoons sweet almond oil, 1 teaspoon wheatgerm oil (borage or evening primrose) with 3 drops each of *tea tree, juniper* and *lavender* (remove excess with cotton wool).

＊ Individual spots can be dabbed with neat *lavender* or *tea tree* (check sensitization first).

＊ A good facial mask can be made by mixing 2 tablespoons of green clay, 2 teaspoons of jojoba oil, 1 teaspoon of yoghurt, with 3 drops each of *juniper* and *cypress* (see page 17).

＊ To help unclog the pores of the skin, put 3 drops each of *cypress* and *geranium* in a bowl of steaming water as a facial steam. Putting *pine needle* oil mixed with water on the stove when having a sauna has a similar effect on the whole body.

＊ 3–5 drops each of *geranium* and *cypress*, OR *juniper* and *rosemary*, OR *petitgrain* and *grapefruit* may be added to the bath water to help detoxify the body. This also acts as a kind of facial steam.

＊ Shaving spots or barber's rash can be helped by the following lotion: 100ml orange flower water and 1 teaspoon vodka to which has been

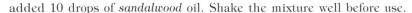

added 10 drops of *sandalwood* oil. Shake the mixture well before use.

✳ Regular massage (by a friend, partner or by a professional), using 3 drops each of *geranium*, *juniper* and *rosemary* in 1 tablespoon basic carrier oil, will also help to stimulate the lymphatic system and rid the body of toxins.

AGEING SKIN, THREAD VEINS AND WRINKLES

Ageing is inevitable, but essential oils can do much to slow down the effects. They encourage regeneration of healthy cells and help to keep the skin supple and elastic. General lifestyle is also, of course, very important, since smoking, drugs, poor diet, too much sun, central heating and stress can all speed up the ageing process.

✳ The regular use of a facial oil containing cytophylactic oils (those that stimulate new cell growth and prevent wrinkles) is vital. They are *lavender*, *neroli*, *frankincense*, *carrot seed*, *myrrh*, *rose* and *patchouli*. Add 3 drops of any of these oils to 1 teaspoon wheatgerm oil, for gentle application, especially to the area around the eyes, before retiring.

✳ A good basic blend for the face and neck is as follows: 1 tablespoon jojoba (or almond) oil, 1 teaspoon wheatgerm oil, 6 drops of *lavender*, 3 drops of *neroli* and 2 drops of *frankincense*. An extra teaspoon of a rich carrier oil such apricot kernel, avocado, hazelnut, evening primrose or peach kernel may also be added.

✳ Gentle facial massage, avoiding the delicate area around the eyes, helps to improve circulation and muscle tone. Use the following blend: 1 tablespoon jojoba (or almond) oil with 9 drops in total of *rose*, *sandalwood*, *jasmine*, *rosewood* or *palmarosa* (or a combination of these).

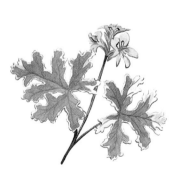

✳ A face mask made by mixing 2 tablespoons clay, 2 teaspoons runny honey, 1 teaspoon water and 4 drops of *rose* oil, used once a week, helps rejuvenation.

✳ Thread veins and broken capillaries are best treated using a facial oil, employing 3 drops of *german chamomile* or *rose* in 1 teaspoon jojoba oil.

DRY AND SENSITIVE SKIN

Dry skin becomes wrinkled more easily than greasy skin and needs to be moisturized regularly, especially when exposed to the effects of central heating or too much sun.

* For a moisturizing treatment for dry skin, add 9 drops in total of *sandalwood*, *geranium* or *ylang ylang* (or a combination of these) to 1 tablespoon of jojoba or apricot kernel oil with 1 teaspoon of a rich oil, such as avocado, borage, evening primrose or wheatgerm, and apply daily. Remove excess with a cotton wool pad.

* A good toner/cleanser for dry skin can be made by adding 5 drops each of *lavender*, *geranium* and *palmarosa* to 75ml rosewater, letting it stand for up to a month before filtering. Then add 25ml glycerine and shake well. Use twice daily.

* For moisturizing sensitive skin, it is important to avoid all possible irritants and to use only the most gentle essences – *roman/german chamomile*, *lavender*, *jasmine*, *neroli* and *rose* are the best choice. Add 5 drops of any of the above oils to 1 tablespoon of jojoba, apricot or peach kernel oil or an anti-allergenic cream or lotion for daily use.

* An excellent basic purifying and rejuvenating face mask for dry and sensitive skin can be made by mixing 2 tablespoons of green clay, 2 teaspoons cornflower, 1 egg yolk, 1 teaspoon evening primrose oil (or other rich vegetable oil) with 1 drop each of *geranium* and *rose* (see page 17). Leave on the skin for 15 minutes, then rinse off with cool water.

ECZEMA (DERMATITIS)

This type of skin condition is characterized by flaky skin, itchy rashes, inflammation and sometimes weeping blisters or scabs. It is frequently associated with hereditary allergic tendences, but often flares up during times of emotional difficulties or stress. It is important to try to locate the cause of the problem and deal with it directly. This means identifying the type of allergens which aggravate the condition and avoiding them (these may be particular household chemicals, dust or certain foods); it may also mean looking at the emotional environment and making changes if necessary.

⁂ In general, the most useful oil for eczema is *roman/german chamomile*. The best medium is usually a non-allergenic light aqueous cream or gel – fatty oils can make the condition worse. Add about 6 drops of *chamomile* to 1 tablespoon of cream or gel to make a very dilute ointment, and apply at least 3 times daily.

⁂ If the condition is weepy or inflamed, 2 drops of *myrrh* or *patchouli* should be included in the above cream or gel.

⁂ If the condition is very itchy, add a few drops of *roman/german chamomile* to a cold compress and apply to the skin. Using a few drops of *chamomile* or *lavender* in the bath can also help to alleviate itching. (A handful of a powdered or colloidal oatmeal, available from some chemists, is also very soothing when added to the bath water.)

⁂ Since eczema takes many forms, and is often stress-related, it is helpful to try to ease emotional tension by using relaxing and uplifting oils such as *benzoin, lavender, geranium, bergamot, neroli* or *rose*, for general use in the bath or as room fragrances.

GREASY AND COMBINATION SKIN

Oily skin is prone to spots and blackheads. It requires careful attention with regard to hygiene, but it is also important not to strip the skin of its protective mantle which maintains the natural PH balance.

⁂ Add 3 drops each of *lavender, bergamot* (bergapten-free – see page 57) and *sandalwood* to 1 tablespoon of a light carrier oil, such as grapeseed or sweet almond oil, and massage into the skin before retiring for the night. (One teaspoon of a nourishing carrier oil may also be included, such as hazelnut, peach kernel, carrot, evening primrose or borage.) Take care to remove all traces of the oil from the face with a tissue or with cotton wool.

⁂ A good toner/cleanser for greasy or combination skin is to mix 5 drops each of *petitgrain, lavender* and *geranium* with 25ml witch hazel and 75ml orange flower water. Let it stand for up to a month then filter. Apply twice daily.

❋ An excellent basic purifying and rejuvenating face mask for greasy and combination skin can be made by mixing 2 tablespoons green clay, 2 teaspoons cornflower, 1 egg yolk, 1 teaspoon evening primrose oil with 1 drop each of *rosemary* and *lavender*. Leave on the skin for 15 minutes, then rinse off with cool water.

❋ Add 5–10 drops of *lemon, palmarosa, rosewood, grapefruit, bergamot, petitgrain* or *geranium* to the bath. This also acts as a facial steam.

HAIR CARE

Since our hair is such a vital feature of our appearance it is important to keep it as healthy as possible. Essential oils can be used in several ways to enhance different hair types.

❋ A few drops (approximately 1 per cent) of an essential oil suited to your hair type can be added to your shampoo – it is always better to use a mild or PH neutral shampoo which does not strip the hair of its protective acid mantle. For greasy hair use *bergamot* or *lavender*; for dry hair *geranium* or *sandalwood*; for fair hair *roman/german chamomile* or *lemon*; and for dark hair *rosemary* or *atlas cedarwood*.

❋ A good rinse for all hair types is to add 5 drops of *rosemary* (or *lavender*) essential oil, together with 1 tablespoon cider vinegar to the final rinse. This will also help to remove detergent residue and restore the acid equilibrium of the scalp.

❋ The following conditioning treatment is excellent for all hair types, but especially if the hair is dry or damaged. Mix 2 tablespoons jojoba oil with 30 drops of an essential oil suited to your hair type. Warm the oil slightly and massage into damp hair, then cover with a shower cap and leave on for 2 hours (if possible). Shampoo out.

❋ Dandruff responds well to *tea tree, rosemary* or *eucalyptus*, used in the shampoo and final rinse. *Patchouli* is also very helpful in the conditioning treatment described above.

❋ An effective tonic, which also promotes hair growth, can be made by

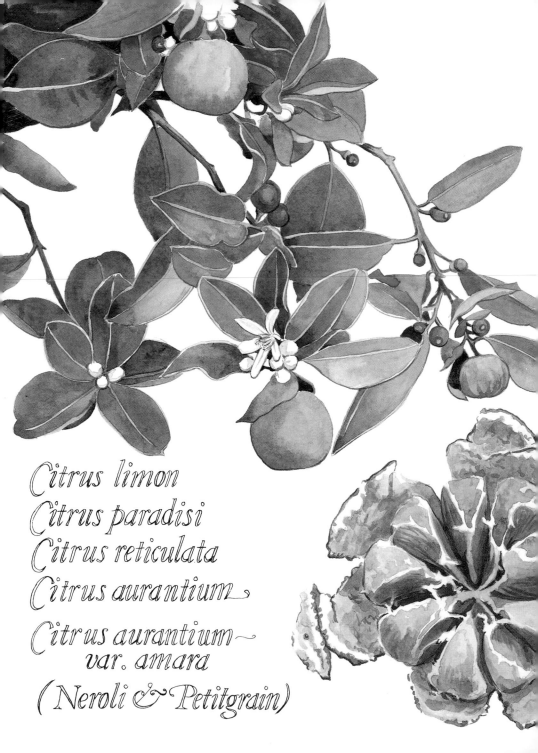

Citrus limon
Citrus paradisi
Citrus reticulata
Citrus aurantium
Citrus aurantium var. amara
(Neroli & Petitgrain)

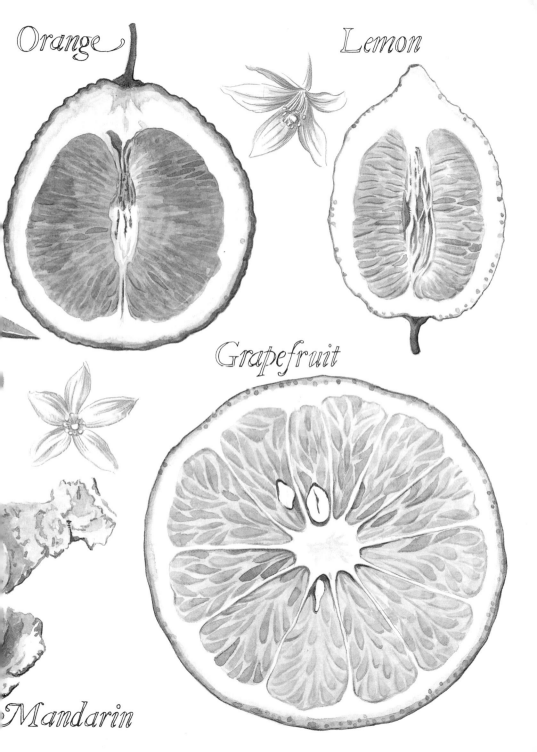

Orange

Lemon

Grapefruit

Mandarin

mixing 1 tablespoon vodka with 5 drops of *rosemary* (or *roman/german chamomile*) and 5 drops of *lavender* and massaging well into the scalp. Other oils which promote hair growth are *spanish sage* and *clary sage*.

✳ Lice is a common problem, especially among school children. *Lavender* and *tea tree* are both very effective in ridding the hair of lice and preventing their return. A few drops (0.5–1 per cent) should be added to a mild shampoo for regular use, and about 5 drops included in the final rinse. In addition, an alcohol-based treatment can be made by mixing 10 drops of *lavender* and 5 drops of *tea tree* with 1 tablespoon of vodka and massaging into the scalp. (If the skin is irritated, use vegetable oil in place of the vodka.)

SKIN CONDITIONS

ABSCESSES AND BOILS

These often occur when the body is exhausted or run down, at times of hormonal upheaval, and especially if the person is on a poor diet. Always keep the area clean, and treat a boil or abscess before it bursts to avoid the spread of infection.

✳ Make up a hot compress using a clean lint with 2 drops each of *tea tree* and *lavender*, and apply to the affected area; then treat it with one drop of neat *lavender* at least 3 times daily if possible. Cover with a plaster only if necessary.

✳ A green clay dressing (see page 68) with 1 drop of *tea tree* may also be used to help draw out the pus.

✳ 5–10 drops of an antiseptic essential oil can also be added to the bath, such as *bergamot*, *roman/german chamomile*, *geranium*, *juniper*, *lavender* or *rosemary*.

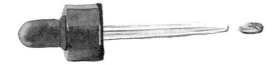

ATHLETE'S FOOT AND RINGWORM

These are both contagious fungal infections characterized by red, flaky skin and itching. Athlete's foot occurs between the toes, sometimes affecting the toenails. Ringworm, which forms a circle on the skin, generally affects the scalp, knees, elbows or between the fingers. Let the skin breathe by avoiding tight clothes and nylon socks.

❋ Make a blend using 1 teaspoon almond oil, 1 drop each of *lavender*, *myrrh* and *tea tree* and apply at least 3 times a day. *Tea tree* may also be applied neat (or diluted in a gel) – check sensitization first by patch test (see page 20).

❋ A few drops of the above oils may also be added to the bath, or to a footbath in the case of athlete's foot.

CHILBLAINS

Chilblains occur at the extremities of the body – fingers and toes mainly – due to cold and lack of circulation. Exercise and warm clothing are important preventative factors.

❋ Apply *lemon* or *tea tree* essential oils neat (or diluted in a gel) to the affected area.

❋ Local blood circulation can be improved by massaging the feet or hands with 2 drops of *marjoram* and 1 drop of *black pepper* in 1 teaspoon carrier oil.

COLD SORES AND HERPES

❋ Mix 3 drops of *tea tree* or *bergamot* (it must be bergapten-free – see page 57) with 1 teaspoon of gel and apply several times daily as soon as the first signs occur.

❋ If the skin keeps cracking, alternate the above treatment with *german chamomile* oil (3 drops in 1 teaspoon wheatgerm oil) or calendula ointment, to keep the area soft.

VARICOSE VEINS AND PILES (HAEMORRHOIDS)

These conditions are both caused by dilated veins brought on by poor circulation and are especially common during pregnancy. Varicose veins occur mainly in the legs; piles or haemorrhoids around the anal area. They both require similar treatments, although sufferers from varicose veins need more patience to see any improvement. The following treatments should be carried out in addition to gentle exercise (inverted yoga postures are especially helpful), keeping weight off the feet as much as possible, improving your diet and losing weight. (See also 'Fatigue, Poor Circulation and Low Blood Pressure', page 33.)

　　* The most useful oils are *cypress* and *geranium*: use 5–10 drops in the bath. Other oils of benefit to use in the bath include *lavender, juniper* and *rosemary*.

　　* To make an oil that will both prevent and alleviate varicose veins, mix 6 drops of *geranium* and 2 drops of *cypress* with 1 tablespoon carrier oil (or add to a non-greasy cream). Then use the oil blend to stroke the legs very gently, working upwards from ankle to thigh (do not massage directly on the veins themselves).

　　* To treat piles, make an ointment by adding 2 drops of *myrtle*, *geranium* or *cypress* to 1 teaspoon of KY jelly, and rub around the anal area as required.

VERUCCAE, WARTS AND CORNS

　　* For these conditions, put a single drop of neat *tea tree* on the centre of the verucca, wart or corn every morning and cover with a plaster. It may take several weeks to see any result – but it is effective in the long run.

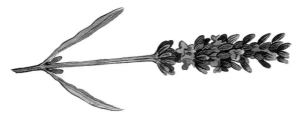

PURELY FOR PLEASURE

Experimenting with the aromatic potential of essential oils can be fun. The oils can be blended in infinite combinations to produce individual perfumes, room fragrances, bath essences, etc. To produce a personal fragrance is also a creative and educational experience.

The different depths of fragrance in a blend are called 'notes', and each scent takes on a particular character according to the balance of base, middle and top notes from which it has been made. Top notes are those light oils which evaporate quickly, like *lemon, bergamot* or *grapefruit*. The middle notes provide the heart of a blend and include oils like *lavender, marjoram* or *rosewood*. The heavier base notes linger for hours, and act as the fixative for the other lighter oils. Traditional base notes are viscous oils like *patchouli, myrrh* and *benzoin*. A well-balanced fragrance should contain elements from each group – top, middle and base notes.

APHRODISIACS

Certain oils have the reputation for increasing sexual desire, including *atlas cedarwood, clary sage, jasmine, neroli, patchouli, rose, sandalwood* and *ylang ylang*. Use 5–10 drops in total of any of these oils (or a combination of them) in the bath, to create a romantic atmosphere.

* Any of the aphrodisiac oils can be burned in a vaporizer in the bedroom to create a sensual mood, or used to scent linen or clothes.

* The spice oils, which include *black pepper, cardomon, nutmeg* and *ginger*, are also reputed to have aphrodisiac properties. However because they are strong stimulants and tend to be dermal irritants in concentration, they should be used only in moderation – 3 drops in the bath or 1–2 drops added to other blends.

✻ The following are recommended sensual massage oil blends: 4 drops each of *rose* and *sandalwood* with 1 drop of *black pepper* in 1 tablespoon carrier oil, OR 3 drops each of *ylang ylang*, *clary sage* and *jasmine* in 1 tablespoon carrier oil.

NOTE Do not let essential oils come into contact with condoms, as they can have a detrimental effect on the rubber.

AROMATIC BATHING

This can be one of the most pleasurable modern-day rituals. It has a long traditional history, and was especially appreciated by the Greeks and Romans. Retire to the bathroom with a few candles and a glass of wine.

✻ Choose 5–10 drops of any essential oil, or a blend of oils, that suits your mood and enjoy an aromatic bath. Always take note of the safety data for each oil (see pages 57–69), avoiding skin irritants or oils which are contra-indicated under certain conditions.

✻ Baths can be used as a gentle way of stimulating the body into action – a good morning bath for hangovers or jet-lag is 5–10 drops of *geranium*, *rose*, *rosemary* or *juniper* (or a combination of these).

✻ A warm aromatic bath is also an excellent way to prepare for a good night's rest. To relax the system after a tiring day, or to combat jet-lag, choose oils such as *clary sage*, *chamomile*, *marjoram*, *lavender* or *vetiver*. Simply add 5–10 drops to an evening bath.

PERFUMES

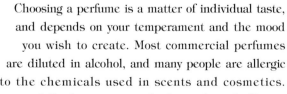

Choosing a perfume is a matter of individual taste, and depends on your temperament and the mood you wish to create. Most commercial perfumes are diluted in alcohol, and many people are allergic to the chemicals used in scents and cosmetics.

✻ For home use it is both simple and effective to wear many essential oils neat as long as you avoid sensitive areas and check your skin reaction first by carrying out a patch test (see page 20).

＊ Alternatively, dilute them to about 5 per cent in jojoba or fractionated coconut oil (which do not go rancid), to make a light oil-based perfume or 'unguent', as used by the ancient civilizations. Dab on wrists and behind the ears.

＊ Sensual, rich or earthy notes include *ylang ylang, patchouli, frankincense* and *vetiver.*

＊ Woody, 'masculine' scents include *sandalwood, cypress, atlas cedarwood* and *juniper.*

＊ Floral, 'feminine' perfumes include *rose, jasmine, neroli* and *lavender.*

＊ Light, refreshing fragrances include *bergamot, geranium, mandarin* and *orange.*

＊ Essential oils such as *lavender* or *rose* can also be used to revive pot-pourris or scent linen, paper or special presents.

ROOM FRAGRANCES

Enhancing the home environment with different fragrances is one of the most traditional uses for aromatics. In medieval times 'strewing' herbs were used to make the house smell pleasant and keep it free of germs. At one time, ladies would provide a different pot-pourri for each room in the house – one scent for the drawing room, another for the bedroom. Incense has been used by all cultures to accompany religious or secular rituals. All sorts of essential oils can be vaporized to get rid of unpleasant odours; to create a fragrance in a room for meditation; to prepare for a party; or to create an intimate mood. Entering into the dimension of fragrance, and learning to blend the oils, can be elevating, relaxing and fun.

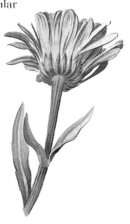

＊ Traditional 'incenses' for meditation, yoga, prayer, etc., include *atlas cedarwood, frankincense, cypress, sandalwood* and *juniper.* Try a few drops of any of these oils (or a combination of them) for use in an oil burner or any other method of vaporization.

✳ Suggested room fresheners, with good antiseptic action, suitable for the kitchen or bathroom, include *bergamot, geranium, pine needle, sweet basil, lemon* or *lemongrass*.

✳ To create a festive mood, make a blend using warm and spicy oils like *orange, cinnamon, coriander* or *nutmeg*. The woody or resinous oils like *pine needle* or *atlas cedarwood* can also be used to enliven the scent of wood intended for burning on an open fire.

✳ Bedroom fragrances may include aphrodisiacs such as *ylang ylang, jasmine* or *clary sage*, or relaxing and soothing scents like *lavender, chamomile* or *geranium*.

✳ Strong penetrating oils like *peppermint* or *basil* are good at dispersing unwanted smells such as cigarette smoke.

✳ Mentally stimulating or cephalic oils, like *rosemary, lemon* or *basil*, can be vaporized in the study or office to increase concentration and help fight fatigue.

✳ Many essential oils are insect repellents and have been used for centuries in this way. *Citronella, lemongrass, atlas cedarwood, lavender, basil, thyme* and *eucalyptus* are some of the most effective – and they give the house a fresh, clean scent.

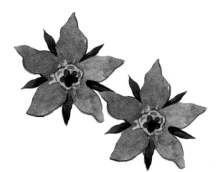

PART THREE

INDEX OF ESSENTIAL OILS

BASIL, SWEET (OCIMUM BASILICUM)

A sweet-spicy essential oil with a clear, refreshing and fortifying scent. An excellent aromatic nerve tonic, which is stimulating to the entire system.

USES: Depression, insect repellent, mental fatigue and poor circulation.

METHODS: Bath (3–5 drops only), massage, vaporizer.

SAFETY DATA: May cause irritation – use in moderation. Avoid during pregnancy; not suitable for babies or infants.

BENZOIN (STYRAX BENZOIN)

A warm, rich essential oil with a comforting vanilla like aroma, well known as an ingredient of Friars Balsam. Good for skin care and respiratory complaints.

USES: Bronchitis, coughs, cuts, depression, eczema, irritated skin and weeping sores.

METHODS: Bath, massage, skin care, steam inhalation, vaporizer.

BERGAMOT (CITRUS BERGAMIA)

A green essential oil with excellent antiseptic properties. It has a strong sedative effect on the nervous system although it has a reviving and uplifting sweet citrus scent.

USES: Abscesses, acne, asthma, boils, cold sores, cystitis, depression, eczema, fever, greasy skin and hair, high blood pressure, mouth and throat infections, pregnancy, spots, stress-related conditions, thrush and whooping cough.

METHODS: Bath, compress, douche, gargle, massage, skin care, vaporizer.

SAFETY DATA: Use only 'bergapten-free' oil for skin care because of the oil's phototoxicity, i.e. it discolours the skin when exposed to direct sunlight.

CARDOMON (ELETTARIA CARDOMOMUM)

A pleasing, warm spicy essential oil with a stimulating effect, reputed to have aphrodisiac properties. Tends to overpower other scents.

USES: Common cold, indigestion and flatulence.

METHODS: Bath (5 drops only), massage, vaporizer.

CARROT SEED (DAUCUS CAROTA)

An amber oil with a warm, woody-earthy odour that has excellent purifying properties. A useful skin care oil.

USES: Ageing skin, arthritis, cellulitis, indigestion, rheumatism, thread veins and wrinkles.

METHODS: Bath, massage, skin care.

CEDARWOOD, ATLAS (CEDRUS ATLANTICA)

A woody-balsamic oil that has a sedative effect, traditionally burnt as an incense and used to repel insects. Good for skin care and respiratory problems.

USES: Anxiety, asthma, bronchitis, coughs, hair care, insect repellent, nervous tension and stress-related conditions.

METHODS: Bath, massage, perfume, skin care, steam inhalation, vaporizer.

SAFETY DATA: Avoid during the first four months of pregnancy.

GERMAN CHAMOMILE (MATRICARIA RECUTICA) AND ROMAN CHAMOMILE (CHAMAEMELUM NOBILE)

German chamomile (or *blue chamomile*) and *roman chamomile* (a yellowy-green oil) share similar properties. They are both excellent sedative and anti-spasmodic oils, though *german chamomile* is a superior anti-inflammatory agent for skin care.

USES: Abscesses, anxiety, arthritis, asthma, boils, bruises, bumps, burns, cold sores, cystitis, dry and sensitive skin, eczema, hair tonic (especially for blonde hair), hayfever, headaches, high blood pressure, indigestion, infected cuts, insomnia, muscular aches and pains, pruritis, rheumatism, scanty periods, sprains, stress-related conditions, sunburn, swellings and thread veins.

These are very 'safe' oils which can be used for a wide range of children's complaints, including chickenpox, nappy rash, restlessness, teething pain and tummy ache.

METHODS: Bath, compress, douche, massage, neat, skin care, vaporizer.

SAFETY DATA: The essential oil *chamomile maroc* is not a true chamomile and does not share the above qualities.

CITRONELLA (CYMBOPOGON NARDUS)

A yellowy-brown essence with a powerful, fresh lemony scent.

USES: Excellent insect repellent.

METHOD: Vaporizer.

SAFETY DATA: May cause an allergic skin reaction in some individuals. Avoid during pregnancy.

CLOVE (SYZYGIUM AROMATICUM)

A pale yellow oil with a strong, sweet-spicy aroma that has excellent antiseptic qualities.

USES: Traditional toothache remedy and gum infections.

METHOD: Apply neat (but do not swallow).

SAFETY DATA: Use in moderation due to toxicity and skin irritation levels. Avoid during pregnancy; not suitable for babies or infants.

NOTE Use only *clove bud* oil – *clove leaf* and *clove stem* oils should not be used at all due to high toxicity levels.

CYPRESS (CUPRESSUS SEMPERVIRENS)

A yellowy-green oil with a sweet, smoky-balsamic fragrance. A good astringent that has a sedative effect on the nervous system. It has been traditionally used as an incense.

USES: Acne, bumps and bruises, cellulitis, greasy skin, heavy periods, oedema, piles, rheumatism, stress-related conditions and varicose veins.

METHODS: Bath, compress, massage, perfume, skin care, steam inhalation, vaporizer.

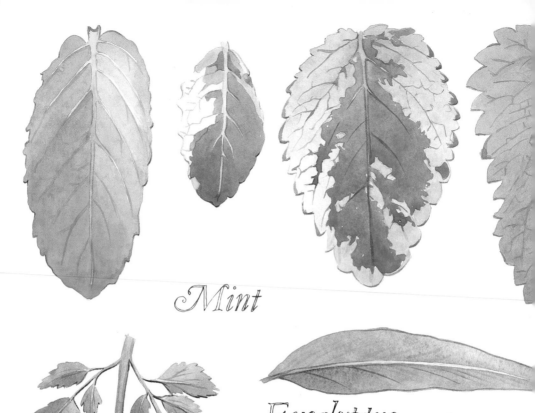

Mint

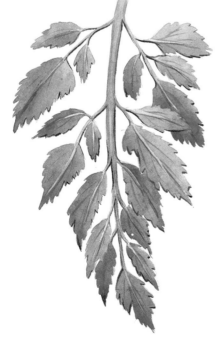

Eucalyptus

Cypress

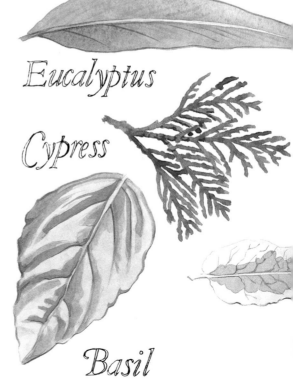

Carrot [wild]

Basil

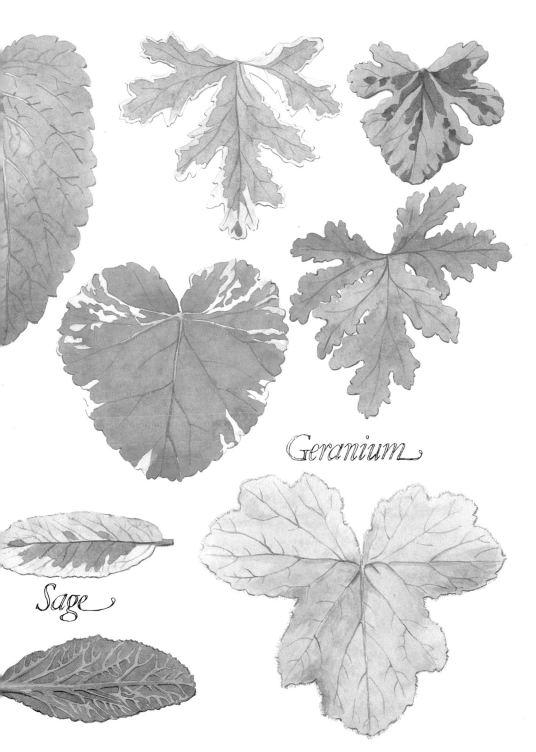

Geranium

Sage

EUCALYPTUS (EUCALYPTUS GLOBULUS)

A clear oil with a strong penetrating (camphoraceous) odour, well known for its decongestant properties. An excellent antiseptic.

USES: Arthritis, bronchitis and coughs, common cold and sinusitis, congested headaches, cuts and sores, dandruff, diarrhoea, fever, flu and infectious illness, insect repellent, muscular pains, rheumatism and whooping cough.

METHODS: Bath (3 drops only), compress, massage, skin care, steam inhalation, vaporizer.

SAFETY DATA: Skin irritant – use in low dilution only. Not suitable for babies or infants; keep away from homeopathic remedies.

NOTE: Eucalyptus oil is toxic if taken internally.

FENNEL, SWEET (FOENICULUM VULGARE)

A pale yellow essential oil with a sweet anise-like scent: a familiar ingredient of gripe water. Good purifying qualities.

USES: Arthritis, cellulitis, indigestion and flatulence, mouth and gum infections, oedema, toxicity and rheumatism.

METHODS: Bath, compress, gargle, massage, skin care.

SAFETY DATA: Use in moderation. Avoid during the first four months of pregnancy; not suitable for babies, infants or epileptics.

NOTE: Bitter fennel oil should not be used at all.

FRANKINCENSE (BOSWELLIA CARTERI)

A pale yellow essential oil with a warm, rich, sweet-balsamic fragrance that has a sedating effect on the nervous system. It helps to calm the mind and is well known as an ingredient of incense. A useful skin care oil.

USES: Ageing skin, asthma, bronchitis and coughs, high blood pressure, scars, stress-related conditions, stretch marks and wrinkles.

METHODS: Bath, massage, perfume, skin care, vaporizer.

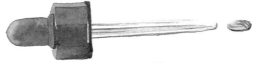

GERANIUM (PELARGONIUM GRAVEOLENS)

A light olive essential oil with a sweet rosy-green scent that has a balancing and harmonizing effect on the nervous system. A good skin care oil.

USES: Acne, anxiety, bumps and bruises, cellulitis, depression, diarrhoea, dry and sensitive skin, eczema, greasy skin, hair tonic, heavy periods, insect repellent, mouth and gum infections, oedema, piles, pregnancy, rheumatism, sore throat, stress-related conditions, sunburn, thrush and varicose veins.

METHODS: Bath, compress, douche, gargle, massage, perfume, skin care, vaporizer.

GINGER (ZINGIBER OFFICINALE)

A yellowy-green oil with a warm, spicy-woody aroma that has a strong stimulating effect on the entire system.

USES: Arthritis, colds, coughs, diarrhoea, indigestion, muscular pain and rheumatism.

METHODS: Bath (3 drops only), massage, steam inhalation, vaporizer.

SAFETY DATA: Use in moderation due to possible skin irritation. Not suitable for babies or infants.

GRAPEFRUIT (CITRUS PARADISI)

A pale yellow essential oil with the fresh, sweet citrus aroma characteristic of the fruit. Good purifying qualities.

USES: Acne, cellulitis, greasy skin, lack of muscular tone, oedema and toxicity.

METHODS: Bath, massage, skin care, vaporizer.

JASMINE (JASMINUM OFFICINALE)

An exquisite perfume oil, with an intense floral fragrance, that uplifts the mind and spirit and has a mildly stimulating effect on the nervous system. An aphrodisiac and useful skin care oil.

USES: Ageing skin, anxiety, depression, dry and sensitive skin, pregnancy and labour, stress-related conditions and wrinkles.

METHODS: Bath, massage, perfume, skin care, vaporizer.

JUNIPER (JUNIPERUS COMMUNIS)

A pale yellow oil with a fresh, woody-balsamic aroma, traditionally used as an incense. Good purifying qualities and is useful for skin care.

USES: Abscesses, acne, arthritis, boils, cellulitis, cystitis, eczema, lack of muscle tone, piles, rheumatism, thrush, toxicity and varicose veins.

METHODS: Bath, compress, douche, massage, skin care, vaporizer.

SAFETY DATA: Use in moderation. Avoid during pregnancy; not suitable for babies or infants.

LAVENDER (LAVENDULA ANGUSTIFOLIA)

A familiar oil with a sweet, floral fragrance and a multitude of uses. It has a marked sedating effect on the nervous system. The most versatile oil of all.

USES: Abscesses, acne, asthma, athlete's foot, boils, bronchitis, bruises, burns and sunburn, cuts, cystitis, dandruff, depression, eczema, hair care, hayfever, headaches, high blood pressure, insect bites and repellent, insomnia, lice, migraine, muscular aches and pains, period pain, PMT, pregnancy, rashes, ringworm, rheumatism, skin care (all types), sores, spots, sprains, stomach ache, stress-related conditions, thrush and varicose veins.

Lavender is a very 'safe' oil, which can be used for a wide range of children's complaints, including chickenpox, nappy rash, restlessness, teething pain and tummy ache.

METHODS: Bath, compress, douche, gargle, massage, neat, perfume, skin care, steam inhalation, vaporizer.

LEMON (CITRUS LIMON)

A fresh, clean-scented citrus oil which has a sedating effect on the nervous system. It has the folk reputation of being something of a 'cure-all'.

USES: Acne, arthritis, chilblains, constipation, cuts, greasy skin, hair care, oedema, rheumatism and toxicity. (Lemon juice is good for sore throats.)

METHODS: Bath (3 drops only), gargle, massage, skin care, steam inhalation, vaporizer.

SAFETY DATA: Skin irritant: do not use *lemon* oil on exposed skin due to its phototoxicity, i.e. it discolours the skin when exposed to direct sunlight. Not suitable for babies or infants.

LEMONGRASS (CYMBOPOGON CITRATUS)

A fresh, grassy-lemon scented citrus oil that has a sedating effect on the nervous system.

USES: Athlete's foot, insect repellent (fleas, lice, mosquitoes, tics), lack of muscle tone, nervous tension and stress-related conditions.

METHODS: Bath, massage, skin care, vaporizer.

SAFETY DATA: Use in dilution only   may cause irritation or sensitization in some individuals. Not suitable for babies or infants.

MANDARIN (CITRUS RETICULATA)

An intensely sweet citrus fragrance, characteristic of the fruit. A mild sedative.

USES: Cellulitis, oedema and stress-related conditions. This oil is especially recommended for children and pregnant women due to its low toxicity level.

METHODS: Bath, massage, skin care, vaporizer.

MARJORAM (ORIGANUM MARJORANA)

A warm, nutty aroma, which has a strong sedating effect on the mind and the nervous system, and a powerful anti-spasmodic action on the muscles of the body.

USES: Anxiety, arthritis, bumps and bruises, chilblains, children's colds and coughs, headaches, high blood pressure, indigestion, insomnia, migraine, muscular aches and pains, period pains, rheumatism and stress-related conditions.

METHODS: Bath, compress, massage, neat, skin care, steam inhalation, vaporizer.

SAFETY DATA: Avoid during pregnancy.

MYRRH (COMMIPHORA MYRRHA)

A rich, warming oil that has been used as a skin remedy for over three thousand years.

USES: Ageing skin, athlete's foot, coughs, cuts, eczema, irritated skin, mouth and gum infections, ringworm, scanty periods, weeping sores and wrinkles.

METHODS: Bath, douche, gargle, massage, neat, skin care, vaporizer.

SAFETY DATA: Avoid during pregnancy.

MYRTLE (MYRTUS COMMUNIS)

A pale yellow oil with a fresh camphoraceous odour, somewhat similar to *eucalyptus* but more pleasing. Reputed to have aphrodisiac properties.

USES: Bronchitis, coughs, flu, piles and respiratory infection. Especially recommended for children's coughs and colds due to its relative mildness.

METHODS: Bath, massage, skin care, steam inhalation, vaporizer.

NEROLI (CITRUS AURANTIUM VAR. AMARA)

An intensely rich, floral perfume, reputed to have aphrodisiac properties. It is uplifting to the mind and spirit but soothing to the nervous system. A useful skin care oil.

USES: Ageing skin, anxiety, depression, dry and sensitive skin, headaches, indigestion, insomnia, PMT, pregnancy, scars, stretch marks, stress-related conditions, thread veins and wrinkles.

METHODS: Bath, massage, perfume, skin care, vaporizer.

NUTMEG (MYRISTICA FRAGRANS)

A warm, sweet spicy oil, well-known as a domestic condiment, that has a sedative effect.

USES: Anxiety, muscular aches and pains, pregnancy (labour) and stress-related conditions.

METHODS: Bath (3 drops only), compress, massage, vaporizer.

SAFETY DATA: Use in moderation due to toxicity levels – narcotic in large doses. Not suitable for babies or infants.

ORANGE (CITRUS AURANTIUM)

A sweet, familiar citrus-scented oil that has a sedating effect on the nervous system.

USES: Oedema, pregnancy, stress-related conditions and tension – good for children's baths.

METHODS: Bath, massage, skin care, vaporizer.

SAFETY DATA: Do not use *orange* oil on exposed skin because of its photo-toxicity, i.e. it discolours the skin when exposed to direct sunlight.

PALMAROSA (CYMBOPOGON MARTINII)

A light olive oil with a sweet, floral rosy-green scent, good for all types of skin.

USES: Ageing skin, dry and sensitive skin, greasy skin and wrinkles.

METHODS: Bath, massage, perfume, skin care, vaporizer.

PATCHOULI (POGOSTEMON CABLIN)

This rich, musky-earthy oil has strong associations with the East, where it is used to scent cloth. It soothes the mind, supports the nervous system and is a potent aphrodisiac.

USES: Ageing skin, anxiety, dandruff, eczema, greasy skin, insect repellent, nervous exhaustion, stress-related conditions, weeping sores and wrinkles.

METHODS: Bath, compress, massage, perfume, skin care, vaporizer.

PEPPER, BLACK (PIPER NIGRUM)

One of the most ancient spices that has been in use for over four thousand years. The pungent, light amber oil has a warming and stimulating effect on the whole system.

USES: Arthritis, cellulitis, chilblains, low blood pressure, muscular aches and pains, nervous exhaustion and fatigue, poor muscle tone and rheumatism.

METHODS: Bath (3 drops only), massage, vaporizer.

SAFETY DATA: Skin irritant – use in moderation in low dilution only. Not suitable for babies or infants; keep away from homeopathic remedies.

PEPPERMINT (MENTHA PIPERITA)

This penetrating, minty oil is cooling and refreshing – it clears the head and revives the spirit.

USES: Asthma, congested headaches, constipation, coughs and colds, fever, flatulent indigestion, flu, insect repellent, mouth and gum infections, muscular aches and pains, nausea and travel sickness, nervous exhaustion and fatigue.

METHODS: Bath (3 drops only), compress, gargle, massage, skin care, steam inhalation, vaporizer.

SAFETY DATA: Skin irritant – use in moderation in low dilution only. Avoid during the first four months of pregnancy; not suitable for babies or infants; keep away from homeopathic remedies.

PETITGRAIN (CITRUS AURANTIUM VAR. AMARA)

A pale yellow oil with a fresh, floral citrus scent – somewhat similar to *neroli*. A classic ingredient of eau-de-cologne.

USES: Acne, greasy skin, nervous tension, oedema and stress-related conditions.

METHODS: Bath, massage, perfume, skin care, vaporizer.

PINE NEEDLE (PINUS SYLVESTRIS)

This fresh, balsamic scented oil is a good antiseptic, with a stimulating and refreshing effect.

USES: Arthritis, coughs and colds, muscular aches and pains, rheumatism and sinusitis.

METHODS: Bath, compress, perfume, skin care, steam inhalation, vaporizer.

SAFETY DATA: Possible skin irritant – use in moderation in low dilution only. Not suitable for babies or infants.

ROSEMARY (ROSMARINUS OFFICINALIS)

A penetrating oil with a warm herbal fragrance and strong stimulating, fortifying properties. A useful skin care oil.

USES: Acne, arthritis, boils and blisters, cellulitis, common cold, constipa-tion, coughs, fever and flu, hair care (dandruff, tonic), low blood pressure, muscular aches and pains, nervous exhaustion and fatigue, oedema, piles, rheumatism, sinusitis and varicose veins.

METHODS: Bath, compress, massage, skin care, steam inhalation, vaporizer.

SAFETY DATA: Avoid during the first four months of pregnancy; avoid if suffering from high blood pressure.

ROSE MAROC (ROSA CENTIFOLIA)

This beautiful feminine scent has long been associated with love. It warms the heart and soothes the nerves. It is especially suitable for children and those with sensitive skin.

USES: Ageing skin, anxiety, asthma and hayfever, depression, dry and sensitive skin, eczema, irritated skin, menstrual problems, pregnancy and childbirth, scars, stress-related conditions, thread veins, thrush and wrinkles.

METHODS: Bath, compress, massage, neat, perfume, skin care, vaporizer.

ROSEWOOD (ANIBA ROSAEODORA)

Also commonly known as Bois de Rose, this oil has a soft woody-floral fragrance, good for rounding off sharp notes when blending. It is a useful skin care oil and is reputed to be an aphrodisiac.

USES: Ageing skin, greasy and combination skin and wrinkles.

METHODS: Bath, massage, neat, perfume, skin care, vaporizer.

SAFETY DATA: The continual use of *rosewood* oil is potentially environmentally damaging as it contributes to the destruction of the rain forests.

SAGE, CLARY (SALVIA SCLAREA)

A pale yellow oil with a pleasing sweet, nutty-herbaceous scent. It is especially good for stress and anxiety states, in comparison to *spanish sage* which is more stimulating.

USES: Anxiety and nervous tension, hair care, labour pain, menstrual irregularity and pain, mouth and gum infections, muscular aches and pains, sore throat, stress-related conditions.

METHODS: Bath, compress, gargle, massage, skin care, steam inhalation, vaporizer.

SAFETY DATA: Avoid during pregnancy; do not use within a few hours of drinking alcohol.

NOTE: It is generally used in preference to *common sage* because of its lower toxicity level.

SAGE, SPANISH (SALVIA LAVENDULAEFOLIA)

A penetrating, stimulating oil with a fresh camphoraceous odour, not as pleasing as *clary sage*. A good antiseptic oil.

USES: Bronchitis and coughs, cellulitis, hair care, measles, mouth and gum infections, muscular aches and pains, poor circulation, sinusitis and sore throat.

METHODS: Bath, gargle, massage, skin care, steam inhalation, vaporizer.

SAFETY DATA: Fairly toxic – use in moderation. Avoid during pregnancy; not suitable for babies or infants.

SANDALWOOD (SANTALUM ALBUM)

This incense, cosmetic and perfume material has enjoyed over four thousand years of uninterrupted use. The oil has a deep, soft woody-balsamic scent which is soothing and very long lasting.

USES: Acne, ageing skin, bronchitis and coughs, depression, dry and sensitive skin, greasy skin, hair care, high blood pressure, nervous tension, stress-related conditions and wrinkles.

METHODS: Bath, compress, massage, neat, perfume, skin care, steam inhalation, vaporizer.

TEA TREE (MELALEUCA ALTERNIFOLIA)

A very useful medicinal oil with a fresh camphoraceous, somewhat offensive, musty odour. It supports the immune system and is active against bacteria, fungi and viruses.

USES: Abscesses and boils, acne, athlete's foot and ringworm, bronchitis and coughs, chickenpox, chilblains, cold sores, common cold, cuts and sores, fever and flu, hair care (dandruff, lice), infectious illness, insect bites, measles, rashes, sore throat, spots, thrush, veruccae, viral infections, warts.

METHODS: Bath, compress, gargle, massage, neat, skin care, steam inhalation, vaporizer.

SAFETY DATA: May cause sensitization in some individuals – do a skin patch test first.

THYME, COMMON (THYMUS VULGARIS)

Thyme oil has a warm spicy-herbaceous odour, with a strong stimulating effect. There are many different 'chemotypes' of *thyme*, depending on their principle constituent – e.g. 'linalol' or 'citral' types which are milder. An excellent antiseptic oil.

USES: Arthritis and rheumatism, bronchitis and coughs, cellulitis, fever and flu, insect repellent, mouth and gum infections, muscular aches and pains and viral infections.

METHODS: Bath (3 drops only), gargle, massage, skin care, steam inhalation, vaporizer.

SAFETY DATA: 'Red' and 'white' *thyme* may cause skin irritation although the 'white' oil is less toxic. Avoid during pregnancy; not suitable for babies or infants; avoid if suffering from high blood pressure.

VETIVER (VETIVERIA ZIZANOIDES)

A dark, viscous oil with an earthy, smoky-woody scent that has a sedating effect on the nervous system.

USES: Anxiety, insomnia, nervous tension and stress-related conditions.
METHODS: Bath, massage, skin care, perfume, vaporizer.

YLANG YLANG (CANANGA ODORATA VAR. GENUINA)

An exquisite perfume oil, with a deep soft floral-balsamic fragrance. It has a marked sedating effect on the nerves, but is uplifting to the spirit – a traditional aphrodisiac.

USES: Anxiety and depression, dry and sensitive skin, high blood pressure, nervous tension and stress-related conditions.
METHODS: Bath, massage, neat, perfume, skin care, vaporizer.

USEFUL ADDRESSES

It is important to buy good quality essential oils for use in the home, if they are to be effective therapeutically. Synthetic perfume oils or diluted products do not have the same potency and cannot be substituted for 100 per cent pure and natural aromatic oils. There are now many brands of essential oils available to the public, but the quality control and ethical standards can vary.

Aqua Oleum has many years' experience in the field and provides a wide range of top-quality essential oils at very competitive prices as well as a large selection of virgin-pressed carrier or base oils. They can be purchased from health and wholefood stores throughout the United Kingdom, as well as from some chemists. Mail order items and further information are available from: Aqua Oleum, Unit 3, Lower Wharf, Wallbridge, Stroud, Glos GL5 3JA. Telephone: 0453 753555.

If you want to experience a professional aromatherapy treatment, it is vital that you choose a therapist who has undergone an accredited training. The International Federation of Aromatherapists ensures that its members have attained a recognized standard of practice and provides a list of qualified practitioners throughout the United Kingdom.

For those wishing to further their interest in aromatherapy, the Federation also publishes a newsletter, holds open meetings and can recommend training programmes for individuals wishing to gain a professional qualification. They can be contacted at: The International Federation of Aromatherapists, Department of Continuing Education, Royal Masonic Hospital, Ravenscourt Park, London W6 0TN. Telephone: 081 846 8066.

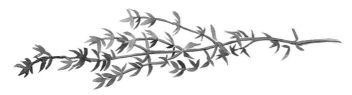

GENERAL INDEX

Page numbers in bold type refer to main entries